# DEMENTIA
# ACTIVIST

Afterword by Dr Elisabeth Stechl and Prof Dr Hans Förstl

# HELGA ROHRA
# DEMENTIA ACTIVIST

## "Fighting for Our Rights"

Jessica Kingsley *Publishers*
London and Philadelphia

First published by Mabuse-Verlag, Germany in 2011
This translation published by Jessica Kingsley Publishers
arrangement with Mabuse-Verlag in 2016
73 Collier Street
London N1 9BE, UK
and
400 Market Street, Suite 400
Philadelphia, PA 19106, USA

*www.jkp.com*

**Library of Congress Cataloging in Publication Data**
A CIP catalog record for this book is available from the Library of Congress

**British Library Cataloguing in Publication Data**
A CIP catalogue record for this book is available from the British Library

ISBN 978 1 78592 071 4
eISBN 978 1 78450 332 1

Printed and bound in Great Britain

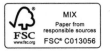

# Contents

> I dedicate this book to everyone affected by dementia, and to the people who are close to them.

# Introduction

My name is Helga Rohra. I am 58 years old, an interpreter, a single mother, and have been living for over three years with a diagnosis of dementia. In this book, I would like to tell you about the way this diagnosis turned my earlier life upside down, the challenges I have had to meet since then, and how I have managed to find new meaning in my life.

But don't worry, my tale is neither a horror story about the "long road to oblivion", nor an account of the trials that come with dementia – quite the opposite.

If you yourself are living with dementia, or notice symptoms in yourself that could be a sign of it, then I would like to share this with you: dementia is not the end! Even with dementia you can have a life of fulfilment, if you come to terms with the disability. I'm not going to paint a rosy picture. Dementia is not child's play and will challenge you every day anew. But one can live with it. Believe me.

If you are close to someone with dementia, or work with people with dementia as a professional or volunteer, I invite you to listen. Perhaps reading this book will help you towards a better understanding of the experiences and needs of people with dementia. But be warned! In a number of my tales about my own experiences, the people providing support to those of us with dementia come in for some mild criticism. Please don't take this as an attack, but try to accept the constructive criticism.

In this book, I am speaking first and foremost for myself, and give an account of my experience as an activist. Other people with dementia have had different experiences, and interpret these in their own ways. My observations make no claim to general validity, although I haven't been able to resist making a few generalisations. It is important for me to draw attention to the special circumstances of younger people with dementia, because the needs of us so-called early onset patients differ not insignificantly from those of older people with dementia. A subject that, in my opinion, is far too little discussed.

I am often asked how my life has changed as a result of dementia, and every time I find it hard to answer, since I have to compare "now" with "then" – and recall, for example, what mattered to me then, and consider whether it still does today. But memories are deceptive, and not just for people with dementia. People without dementia also have to ask themselves honestly whether their recollections reflect the truth. They too emphasise their successes, consciously or unconsciously, and overlook their failures. Every time we tell a story the narrative deviates somewhat from the previous version, because a story from the past is always told in light of, and against the background of, the present. So even "normal" memories undergo a certain transformation. Dementia makes remembering more difficult. For me, the past is no longer the rock on which today is built. Memories are often more like a treacherous swamp – here firm and safe, but over there perilous and unstable, swallowing things up and unexpectedly releasing them again. So the answer to the question about what changes dementia has made to my life is always a current one. That is to say, it depends on what I remember at the time. For this reason I need to explain to you how this book came about.

I would like to tell you that my editor and publisher offered me the book project, whereupon I enthusiastically agreed, sat down at my desk and eagerly started writing. Unfortunately, it was not that simple. It's true that I was asked if I would like to tell about my experiences as a person with dementia, but I couldn't simply go off and write. Easy as it is for me to tell the story and talk about my experiences, I find writing long pieces difficult, especially ones about my own experiences. Dementia deprived me of this ability.

It has made calling up memories so tiring that I can no longer write them down. So how were my spoken words and brief notes to become the text that you now hold in your hands in book form? The simplest solution would have been a ghostwriter, such as takes on the writing of many an autobiography, but remains hidden as a person. However, this way of doing things was not on – for me, the editor or the publisher. It wouldn't do to create the impression that I had written the book by myself from beginning to end.

My partner on this book is Falko Piest. He himself would describe his role as that of writing assistant – a role that he took on once before, in another book project to which I also contributed. We met in 2009 and together wrote my chapter in *Ich spreche für mich selbst: Menschen mit Dementia melden sich zu Wort* [*Speaking for Myself: People with Dementia in Their Own Words*], which appeared under my pseudonym of Helen Merlin. Since then we have written several articles together as a practised team, and have repeatedly appeared at events. Falko Piest is deeply involved professionally with the person with dementia's point of view. As a research associate of "Dementia Support Stuttgart" he devotes himself enirely to the participation and self-expression of people with dementia.

For the purposes of the present book Falko listened to me for many hours, with lots of questions and discussion. This text eventually emerged from the recordings we made of our conversations, together with my own notes and diary entries – not in one piece and not in chronological order, but one chapter at a time. Every time an episode had been written up, he sent me the text to comment on and say what I would like to change. A bit at a time, it turned into a complete book.

# ONE

# Prior to the first symptoms

I was born on 19 March 1953 as Helga Anneliese Schuller, in Siebenbürgen, Romania, where I grew up and went to school. As a member of the German minority in Romania at that time, in 1972 I emigrated with my parents and two brothers to Germany, where, to begin with, we were accommodated in a reception camp near Nuremberg. After that we very quickly moved in with my mother's sister in Munich. One of my first memories of Munich is of the 1972 Olympic Games, which at the time enthralled the entire city. The cosmopolitan flair, the freedom and apparently unlimited opportunities exceeded everything that I had experienced in Romania. It was natural for me to want to be independent as soon as possible and stand on my own two feet, if only to get away from the cramped conditions at my aunt's. More than anything I would have liked to study medicine, but my Romanian school-leaving report was not recognised as equivalent to the German *Abitur* [school leaver's examinations], and so

I looked for an alternative. As I had been fascinated by foreign languages since childhood, and had grown up bilingual, I decided to train as an interpreter. At the first opportunity I registered at the Language and Interpreting Institute in Munich, which accepted my Romanian educational status. I studied English, with natural sciences as my main subject and French and Italian as subsidiary subjects. All that I still lacked was a flat of my own. There were no rooms to be had in the student halls of residence, but by means of a newspaper advertisement I found a position as an *au pair* with an industrialist family. Thus I had free board and lodging and, in addition, more than generous pay – even the cost of obtaining my driving licence was paid for me.

Directly after the state examination I found a job teaching at a school for foreign language correspondents in Waldkraiburg, where my parents now lived. A nice challenge, it must be said, for a brand new graduate, but, much as I enjoyed teaching, I felt that I was not being stretched as a linguist and so, as a sideline, I began interpreting for businesses.

After a brief and unhappy marriage, I divorced my first husband, which in provincial Bavaria in the 1970s was positively scandalous. So as not to constantly keep having to justify myself for getting divorced, I left Waldkraiburg and went back to Munich. There I began getting established as a freelance interpreter. On one of my commissions, a guided tour of a Munich brewery,

I met my second husband, Volker Rohra, who at that time was a teacher.

Sadly, our marriage broke up when our son Jens was starting the second year at school, and I left my husband the house we jointly owned. Jens and I moved into a small flat on the outskirts of Munich, where we still live now. For Jens the move was difficult. A few months previously he had been diagnosed with Asperger's Syndrome, a mild form of autism, because of which he had a particular need for reliability and a stable environment. For me it was the beginning of a time of precise planning and organisation. As I wanted to be financially independent from my ex-husband and make my own living, I had to coordinate my interpreting work very carefully with my son's time at school. Sometimes I simply took him with me, which he enjoyed, and my clients mostly didn't mind.

Although our daily routine was very structured and my work often began at 6.00am and went on late into the evening, I was happy with my life. The days were filled with activities, and minutely planned appointments and tasks kept me on my toes. Languages were my life, and I could think of nothing nicer than to be working freelance. Every day brought new challenges, and I rejoiced at being able to give my best. When I wasn't interpreting I taught students and coached schoolchildren. Depending on my work situation I sometimes translated from English, French or Romanian. Like other interpreters, I also had my specialisms, with the main emphasis on medicine and medical research, because I was very interested in this subject matter. So I frequently enjoyed taking part in medical training sessions. In particular, the human brain, with its huge capacity for performance and adaptability, fascinated me. It is an irony of fate that a thorough training in caring for people with dementia was once part of my training programme.

I particularly enjoyed working with the young people whom I taught. I enjoyed engaging with schoolchildren, and tried to recognise their strengths and develop them in an appropriate way. The children were evidently happy with me, since word-of-mouth referrals were sufficient to keep me busy.

It always mattered to me to be in touch with people. I wanted to create harmony and I drew my inner strength from the respect of others, their praise and my faith. I don't know whether I am a religious person; for one thing, I'm not a regular churchgoer. Even so, I have always found energy and inner strength in prayer and meditation. Far be it from me to try to convince others of my views, but I have to mention that I believe in God, because this has been, and remains, an important source of strength in my life, and I am also convinced that without it I would not today be in a position to tell of my experiences.

When I write about all this it brings home to me how different my life is today. Was it me, who once had that life? And I feel infinite wistfulness, but also, at the same time, pride.

In spite of everything, with or without dementia, I am still here!

# TWO

# Summer 2008: There's something the matter with me

It took a while for me to become aware that something was the matter with me. There was nothing concrete by which to identify it, but rather the sum of many little peculiarities that caught my attention.

On many days my structured programme was too much for me, and I was having difficulty concentrating and working systematically. To begin with I thought it was exhaustion, which I explained to myself was due to the workload of my multi-tasking job. That alone was not yet cause for concern. Then I noticed increasingly often that when I was translating from one foreign language into another, certain vocabulary would no longer come to me spontaneously – an unusual situation for me, as here I could normally work very rapidly. It was frustrating for me to experience limitations in a competence that was the reason for getting work as an interpreter.

The last job that I can still remember clearly was an international medical conference on multiple sclerosis at the beginning of 2008. During the event everything had gone smoothly and the client was satisfied. About a week after the conference the organisers offered me a follow-up task: the conference papers were to be translated. I would gladly have taken on the job, but I felt stunned: I couldn't think what I had translated at that conference. Everything seemed to have been wiped out, yet I had worked for days to master the vocabulary. "It can't be that you can't remember anything any more," I told myself, but it made no difference. On the pretext that I had no time, I recommended a colleague. Out of shame and fear of recourse I was unable to tell the truth. After all, the organisers could have taken the line that "If she can't remember the conference topics any more, who knows what Mrs Rohra's interpreting was about?"

Additional symptoms occurred with increasing frequency. For example, in mid-sentence I would begin to pick the wrong words. I would intend to say "Look, here comes *der Hausherr* [the owner of the house]" – but what I said was: "Look, here comes *die Haussocke* [the slipper sock]." I was no longer able to name certain things – "What do you call the thing that salt comes out of?" "Oh God," I thought to myself, "what fun it's going to be if slips of the tongue like these happen in the wrong places!" To begin with, my son and I would laugh about it, and we began writing down what we called "these pearls".

On the one hand I treated it humorously and blamed it on tiredness. On the other hand it was an entirely new, scary situation for me. My friends, people who knew me well, and had done for years, said that I suddenly started talking in a laborious way, but they would also say, "It's somehow like you, because you always like to talk in a roundabout way." But if, in conversations with them, I didn't immediately grasp certain connections, or replied to a question in a way that didn't make sense, I might hear: "How dumb can you be!" Only my son would pat me on the back and say, "Look here, you need to rest more."

Without work, I was at home more and more often, and for longer. When Jens was out, at school or sports activities, a great sadness came over me. I felt incapable of doing any kind of work. It wasn't just the uncertainty about what was wrong with me, but also the lack of energy and the feeling of being quite unable to think properly. After a while I decided to chat with friends on the internet in order to offload my worries. I sat at my laptop and just about managed to switch it on. "But now what, what's my password?" It was all gone.

I wouldn't give up: "You can't throw in the towel just like that. Turn off the laptop, get out into the open, the light, and when you get back, try again." But it made no difference. I tried again several times, but in vain! The laptop, at which I had worked for so many hours, was now nothing more than an overpriced paperweight. I tried to conceal from my son the fact that I was incapable of doing anything on the PC. I merely said, "Jens, I've forgotten so many things!" He replied, "No, you just can't remember them at the moment. You'll see!"

After turning down the follow-up job from the MS conference, I also stopped taking on any other work. My son noticed this, of course, and asked, "Why are you turning everything down, you've got plenty of time, haven't you?" I replied that at the moment I was feeling overloaded. He responded very sympathetically and advised me to take time for myself and rest. Luckily he didn't think of the financial consequences, as that would have been certain to weigh heavily on his mind.

From then on he wrote my emails and took over everything on the PC. He relieved me of many other tasks as well. He did the shopping, reminded me about important things, and generally kept an eye on things. My activities became ever more limited. I was still just about able to have breakfast with Jens. Around midday I would force myself to get up off the sofa and go out, at least for half an hour. It was a very bad time. In fact, all I did was cry and ask myself the same questions over and over again: "What is it? If only I knew. Is it the effect of a trauma? Or maybe I have a brain tumour that's pressing on certain areas."

The symptoms kept getting worse. If I walked a bit further than usual, beyond my own neighbourhood, I couldn't recognise my own street when I got back. Can you imagine how it feels, having to ask yourself: "Is this the way I came just now? Where do I live now?" I still knew my address and kept encouraging myself: "Just ask a passer-by which way it is, then walk a bit further and ask again." That way I eventually managed to get home each time.

As I go into such detail about the difficulties I was having at that time, maybe you are getting the impression that every day was simply dreadful – but it wasn't quite as devastating as that. On many days my memory would work quite well, and my sense of direction was not always consistently bad. But on days when the symptoms were more obvious, I was mostly very depressed. It got to the point where I was really lethargic. Then everything was simply too much for me. Making a cup of coffee in the morning – impossible. A glass of tap water will do. Housework, tidying, cleaning, laundry – unthinkable. You can imagine what it looked like in my flat. On days like that, most of all I would have liked to crawl under the bedclothes with a bottle of whisky. Had it not been for my son and my responsibility towards him, I believe I would have let myself go completely. But because of him I had a reason to keep going, and I had to pull myself together as best I could.

One day I made the effort to tidy up our cellar, so that my enforced break from work was at least being put to good use. When I came out of the cellar area I felt as if I was on an alien planet. In our block of flats you have to go round a few corners and down long corridors to reach your part of the cellar, but I don't believe that even a child could get lost there. Although I must have made my way from the cellar to the lift some few hundred times in the past few years, on this day I couldn't find it straight away. I was gripped by an oppressive feeling, I could feel panic rising inside me. "If the light goes off now…" I imagined. Fear clutched my chest until I thought I couldn't breathe. My heart was thumping madly. After what felt like an infinity, I finally found the door of the lift. Bathed in sweat and with my nerves in tatters, I pressed the button for my floor. Fortunately I still knew which one it was.

A few days later something very odd happened. I started seeing a film in front of me. The images were in colour, scenes from my youth. Images that I didn't even know existed. They appeared in rapid succession, without any connection to what I was doing, seeing, or who I was talking to. No matter whether I was making myself a coffee in the kitchen, talking to a neighbour, or watching television – this film was with me all the time.

It was there at night too, so that I wasn't sure: "Am I asleep now, dreaming, or am I watching the film?"

Of course I was afraid: "Am I going crazy?" In my entire family no one, as far as I could remember, had ever had mental health or psychiatric problems. "What's happening to me?" I avoided all phone calls, declined invitations. I needed time to reflect on all these changes. In the end I reached a decision.

# THREE

# Summer 2008:
# First consultation with the
# doctor – "Go for walks"

So in summer 2008 I went to a neurologist/psychiatrist, simply to one whose consulting rooms I could easily get to. Naturally, having finally made up my mind, I wanted an appointment straight away. Faced with the receptionist, I insisted vehemently that I was an emergency case. She replied, "Everyone is an emergency here. The first free appointment is in three weeks." Another three weeks of waiting – it was too much for me. The defences that I had built up around myself in recent weeks broke down. In tears, I entreated her: "I can't stand any more, I'm at rock bottom." Maybe she had noticed that I really was very unwell. Possibly she just wanted to put an end to the scene. At any rate, I was allowed to take a seat in the waiting room. After a while it was my turn. I told the doctor about my symptoms, the word-finding difficulties, my disorientation, all my cognitive limitations, my optical hallucinations and my deep depression. I also mentioned that I worked freelance, and appealed to the doctor: "I need urgent help. You see, I'm on my own, responsible for myself and my son. If I can't work, I'm ruined." I was just about able to speak coherently and I absolutely had to know what was the matter with me. The doctor listened to it all, and in the end he said, "You've got burnout syndrome. With a demanding job like yours, it's no wonder. I advise you to take time out for three months, and then come back." To which I replied, "Doctor, if that's what you say – I will trust you. But could you at least give me something to help with my depression, to give me a bit of strength?" He replied, "Just go out for walks, there's nothing else you need."

So with that advice I went home. I was somewhat sceptical, but I tried to convince myself: "The doctor must know best!" Weeks passed and there was no improvement. Although there was no shortage of inquiries, I couldn't take on any work. I was simply in no position to work. My son had to cover up for me. Under no circumstances did I want anyone to find out how I was.

I hadn't asked for a sick note – what was the point? Unfortunately, as a self-employed person, I had no sickness insurance in place. So I drew on my financial reserves and tried to build myself up through meditation, going for walks and a healthy diet. I sought in prayer the strength to keep being a strong mother to my son. I knew and sensed that right now, with so little time left before the *Abitur*, he needed encouragement. Divulging my innermost fears, and my visit to the doctor, would (I believe today) surely have undermined him and sapped his strength. He had such great plans. He wanted to sign on with the army for a career as an officer. He had tests and assessments ahead of him. He needed his energy. And I saw myself as being responsible for supporting my son.

The weeks passed, and then came Christmas 2008 – and with the Christmas season came the many thoughts and memories of lovely, happy times with my family. When my parents were still alive, when my ex-husband, my son and I were in our wonderful house with the open hearth. Was I sad about what was lost and gone? Was I afraid of what my next Christmas was going to be like? I felt worse and worse. On top of my mental and spiritual problems I had physical symptoms: weight loss, high blood pressure, heart problems, stomach and intestinal problems. My strength was dwindling. The only thing I wanted was to lead a normal life, just like it had been before. I began writing my symptoms down in a kind of diary. I made a note of everything – my lapses, with the precise time; when I made phone calls or when I had visitors; and everything I had said, and that had been said to me.

And then in 2009, in January, I went back to the neurologist and told him about my condition. I had my so-called "deficit diary" with me. I told him that I wasn't feeling any better. "Even my body is feeling ill. Since last time, I've lost over 10kg. My lapses, my hallucinations. Somehow I have the feeling that everything has got worse, and I've even kept a record of it, here, in my handwriting, in my diary. What am I to do next? What's the matter with me?"

And this expert, the good consultant neurologist, with his expensive training and years of experience – what was the outcome of his assessment? Well, no one could accuse him of giving complicated advice: "Take more time out, keep going for walks for a few months longer," he said. And still no concrete suggestion of therapy, no medication. I left, unable to swallow not only my tears, but my rage. He had told me nothing, not even an approximate explanation of my deficits. He just wasn't taking me seriously.

Even today, a full three years later, I hold him responsible. Without a doubt, a diagnosis of dementia, especially in younger people, is a tricky business. No serious doctor would give a diagnosis of dementia lightly. And yet I am convinced that, had I been not in my mid-fifties, but in my late sixties at the time, the full arsenal of diagnostic procedures for dementia would have been open to me. But at the time I went home furious and disappointed, and thought about his advice. In prayer, I sought a way forward. I had no one I could or wished to talk to about it. Yes, I wanted to go this way on my own, wanted certainty, for myself.

# FOUR

# Why is early onset dementia so late in being recognised?

At the risk of repeating myself, but by all means put it down to my dementia if I do, people with dementia are generally imagined to be old, disorientated and totally reliant on others. In broad swathes of the population, dementia is viewed from the end point. The dominant picture in people's minds is the impression of the final stages, frequently overlooking the fact that at some time dementia also has a beginning. Alzheimer's and Lewy Body dementia begin slowly, insidiously, their symptoms being difficult to distinguish from other illnesses. The first symptoms, such as difficulty remembering and problems with orientation, can be caused just as much by other illnesses such as depression, burnout syndrome, mental illnesses or metabolic disorders – which doesn't exactly make diagnosis easy. A further diagnostic problem lies to this day in the fact that for many forms of dementia there are no direct diagnostic procedures. Neither Alzheimer's nor Lewy

Body can be determined with certainty using imaging techniques, blood tests or the like. For this reason the initial pathway to diagnosis involves eliminating all other diseases that can cause similar symptoms. Lewy Body dementia and also Alzheimer's are, so to speak, residual diagnoses, left over when everything else has been ruled out. Hence, a diagnosis of dementia is never 100 per cent certain, but applies only with some degree of probability. Diagnosis is made easier if the symptoms are precisely described, according to my current doctor, who was very glad of my detailed recording of symptoms; some of my symptoms, in particular optical hallucinations, can be a clear indicator of Lewy Body dementia.

It's often said that the greatest risk factor for getting dementia is age, and the statistics also show this. In 65 to 69-year-olds the risk is about one per cent; in the over-90s, over one third of people are diagnosed. In my age group, the under-60s, the risk is very, very small. But what good is a slight risk of illness if you have got dementia? None at all. Worse still, the doctors don't have a disease of this sort on their diagnostic radar, and so diagnosing it, as happened with me, can take a long time.

You may be asking yourself: "What's the point of a diagnosis that, first, is uncertain; second, takes a long time; and third, represents the end of an illness for which there is virtually no treatment?" An entirely justifiable question, and I can understand people with memory problems not wanting to subject themselves to this process. People who perhaps want to avoid the label "dementia" because they fear being degraded and excluded as a result of the stigma. Counter to this argument one could say that in the course of the diagnostic process a treatable illness might be recognised, the symptoms of which it might be possible to deal with, even if the ultimate diagnosis turns out to be dementia.

In retrospect I am glad to have a diagnosis, and thus certainty. I now know what is wrong with me, can classify my symptoms, and address the dementia. This also means that I am better able to live with my disabilities. If, for example, I can't concentrate, I know now that it's not just because of my lack of willpower, but because of the changes in my brain. This insight relieves me of a heavy burden.

But back to the problems of younger patients, sometimes referred to as "early onset" patients (giving rise to some degree of uncertainty as to which patient group is meant). Mostly, those called early onset patients are those whose dementia began at a younger age, say before their 65th birthday. To an extent, it is also taken to mean people in the beginning of dementia-related changes, independent of age. I count myself as one of the early onset group, because in me the first symptoms were appearing as early as in my mid-fifties, and I am convinced that I am still in the beginning stage of dementia.

In my opinion, whether the symptoms begin when they are young, or not until a more advanced age, makes a big difference for patients. I don't mean to say that dementia is worse per se for a young person than it is for an older one. The impact of dementia shattering patients' lives may well be no less great, whatever our age. Nevertheless, for those of us in the early onset group there are different questions and things to get to grips with, since our life circumstances differ markedly from those of older people.

There is, first, the problem of social perception: apparently youth and dementia don't go together. Further, the relatively small early onset patient group is less visible, and for that reason there is less awareness of it. Consequently, society also knows little about our needs and problem areas, which, not least, explains the scant number of opportunities on offer specifically for early onset patients.

I cannot speak for all early onset patients, but nevertheless my situation is comparable with that of many others. Dementia snatched me away from my career at a time when retirement was still a long way off, and this brought significant restrictions with it.

If I had already been retired, I would have been sure to be spared from the spectre of state benefits. Today I receive a reduced earnings capacity pension, which is not enough to live on, so that I am also reliant on housing benefit. I have no money left to put aside for care in old age, and I have been obliged to use up most of my savings. When, at age 65, I can draw my state pension, I shall be short of a number of years' contributions. In other words, there is little prospect of improvement in my financial position, even with the state pension. It's a situation that I have in common with many people who have had to give up their occupation prematurely, whether they have dementia or not. With dementia, the mandatory business with the authorities certainly becomes very difficult – especially as most of the application forms ask questions about aspects of the past which I can often no longer remember; and not infrequently I have also forgotten where the relevant documents – insurance policies, evidence of earnings, birth certificate, etc. – are. First of all there is the effort of finding everything, which makes it not always easy to meet official deadlines. A further problem that many early onset patients struggle with is the situation of their own children, if they are not yet able to stand on their own two feet. My son is still in the middle of further education, and won't foreseeably complete his studies for another two or three years. At the moment he is busy finding his own way. Why should he also have to worry about his mother, whose dementia could take a completely unpredictable course?

In many respects society is not yet attuned to the difficulties that those of us with early onset dementia, be it the employment services or the integration services that are ill-prepared for dealing with people with dementia, or the employers, who are unwilling to keep on people in the initial stages of dementia, and are mostly not prepared to consider the competencies and resources that we have in spite of our disability. The welfare organisations, too, with their charitable institutions, are still in the early days when it comes to developing any assistance to offer to us. Most of what's on offer for people with dementia is focused around care and help for the elderly and, if only for that reason, is unattractive to most people with early onset dementia. We aren't elderly, and don't feel it either. We are in the middle of life!

What we lack is an advocacy group to represent our interests, through which to raise our concerns at the local as well as the higher political level. Of course, there are the Alzheimer's societies who intervene on behalf of us. I myself have been elected to the executive board of the Munich Alzheimer's Society. But still, in my opinion, we are not yet adequately represented on social committees. It's not enough for organisations to wait until individuals themselves take action – rather, they should be actively on the lookout for people with dementia, and involving them in committee work. We early onset patients, who are still in the middle of our lives, still have loads of abilities and knowledge that we would gladly offer – by volunteering, too – to help improve the lives of everyone with dementia, if only we were allowed to.

# FIVE

# Spring 2009: At the University Health Centre – Waiting and hoping

At the beginnning of 2009 I set off for the memory clinic at the Munich University Health Centre. Normally it takes months to get an appointment here. However, desperation gave me strength, and I got my way. "It's my life, I'm entitled to see an expert who will take my symptoms seriously, straight away." And, just imagine, I was seen without delay. Maybe someone took pity on this woman, sitting there waiting in a heap of misery. In the waiting room, as a matter of fact, there were only couples. I felt very small, so alone, so desperate. But I was certain that this was the way I had to go. I needed certainty.

The tests lasted all day and took place in a protected unit, once called a "closed unit". Here, the laboratory tests were done: spinal cord puncture, CT, MRI, and so on and so forth. A battery of tests was on the programme, the usual ones for Alzheimer's (as I later discovered). Then I had to tell my entire life story, from my childhood up to the present. It was all very exhausting for me. In the end I could scarcely go on, and the doctor suggested that I stay in as an inpatient.

But I could see the other patients, most of whom gave the impression of being very disturbed; and the locked door that needed a special code to open it. I was scared. I wanted to decide for myself where and when I spent my time. So I said that I would be prepared to come back the following day to have further tests and the concluding talk with the senior doctor and the team. I signed a statement to say that I had declined to stay on the ward. "And, yes, I'm coming back. No, I don't need to be escorted. After all, I got here by myself."

I suppose that in the memory clinic they were accustomed to every patient who came for this consultation having somebody with them. I had always been an independent person, and I wanted to take the path to my diagnosis on my own too, without any companion. How did I spend the night, are you wondering? How well did I sleep? Well, actually, it was more of a floundering around in my hallucinations. I was restless, repressing my fear, and hoping: "No, it can't be anything bad. Maybe it really is just burnout." But the next minute I went back to being realistic: "Those aren't the symptoms of burnout." I developed a strategy: "No matter what it is, I want to know. I'll start doing something about it straight away. I have confidence in my body. I can handle anything."

So the next day I went resolutely back to the clinic. They did more tests, and then it was a matter of waiting...

Have you ever had to wait for a diagnosis? Have you ever sat, with no one for support, in a waiting room with people in tears, and the scent of the end of life in the air, where you have a sense of eternal dusk?

But it returned, that strength; I had a strong sense of rejecting any end, of whatever sort. I wanted daybreak. Before me I saw the work I had to do, both professional and private. So many plans. I still felt very young in comparison to the elderly people sitting in the waiting room. I grounded myself, summoned up my strength, and was ready for THAT talk.

In the room sat several doctors, the consultant and a psychologist. I felt as if I was in front of an examination board. I felt dizzy – everything even looked a bit blurred. Once more my results were analysed, opinions aired about key events in my life, my lifestyle discussed. "Yes, all right – but what's wrong with me, why these deficits, it can't be normal?" Saying that the team had to give it further consideration, they were about to send me away. The final verdict would be sent to my neurologist. "Oh, no. No more waiting," I thought to myself. But at the same moment, reason kicked in: "All my neurologist did was tell me to go out walking. No, he's not going to treat me." So I asked the clinic for a referral.

They referred me to a nearby group practice. I marched off there and told the receptionist that the clinic would be sending my results within the next few days. Then, yet again, it was a case of dragging myself home, struggling, putting on an act, trying not to give anything away, and hoping.

At last came the day that I had been waiting for for so long. I went briskly, and on my own, to the neurology practice where my results had been sent from the memory clinic at the University Health Centre. I handed in my card at the reception desk and said briefly, "I'm expecting results from the clinic." The receptionist took €10 from me and showed me into the waiting room. The waiting room was full. Young and old, some with a companion. No conversation; an unusual silence reigned. I sat down on a chair from where I could see everyone else. The fear, the uncertainty, the helplessness were palpable. I could see all the doctors as they called the patients in, one after another. One of them made me think to myself: "I hope this frantic fellow isn't the doctor who's treating me." Waiting; minutes seemed an eternity, time frozen. I wasn't thinking about anything. I felt lifeless, timeless, as if I were waiting for a life sentence!

And then there was an elderly doctor standing in front of me. He seemed very calm and serious. He asked me to follow him into his consulting room. Holding a few sheets of paper, he gave me a searching look. I was sitting in front of him on a chair with an enormous backrest, which made me feel even smaller. My first question was: "Doctor, what do the results say? Which way is it going with me?" Somehow, I felt certain. "I can't have Alzheimer's," I thought. "I'm much too young for that." He looked at me hard and began, "I think it's something that's quite uncommon. But I'd like to make sure and wait for another test." He didn't tell me what I had, but referred me to a radiologist.

More waiting. Another medical appointment. "What's all this?" I said to myself, and a few days later underwent some scan or other. After the test I asked the radiologist if he could tell me what was the matter with me. "Oh, don't worry, it's nothing. It's just depression," was his encouraging reply. The results, he said, would go to my neurologist. I left the practice feeling mentally stronger, assuming that now I had a reliable diagnosis.

The next day I called at the neurologist's, hoping to be able to begin treatment at last. He opened the conversation by asking if the radiologist had told me anything about the diagnosis. I said yes, and smiled at him.

Without reacting to my smile, he said, "What you've got is Lewy Body dementia."

# SIX

# The diagnosis:
# I feel as if I'm falling

After the doctor gave me my diagnosis, just like that – he can have had no idea that the radiologist had spoken to me of depression – I felt as if I was falling. I saw myself on a slide that descended precipitously into a black tunnel, down and down… I began to cry. Now, as I write about it, this feeling comes back. As if I could skid away again at any moment. I want something to hold onto – but what, or whom?

A spark of hope stirred in me. "Doctor, your colleague told me something quite different." But his judgement was final: "Look, here it is in writing." Without thinking, automatically, I demanded to see a copy of the results, and received it without further ado. Even today, I still can't understand how I was able to act so rationally at that moment. I asked, "Doctor, what's going to happen to me? What can I do?" Instantly came the answer: "Well, you should consider a general power of attorney, perhaps draw up a living will."

Inwardly, without further reflection, I rejected this suggestion. I immediately associated the idea of giving anyone power of attorney with "the-end-is-nigh", and I would not allow that thought. I suppose I was afraid that being mentally preoccupied with the end of the illness might paralyse me. And of course, I didn't want to give up my independence by placing myself in someone else's hands – although, as I now know, setting up a general power of attorney is not about giving up autonomy. But that was how it appeared to me at that moment. Then, a few days later, it occurred to me that I didn't even *have* anyone to appoint as an attorney. Only one person could be considered as someone I trusted unreservedly. My son alone was close enough to me to take on this role; but I didn't want to burden him, especially, with this enormous responsibility.

The doctor then showed me out of the consulting room with the following words: "And look, here's a leaflet for you. The people there will be a support for you. Ring them up. If you're feeling better, come back in a day or two and get some medication."

I have no idea how I got from the consulting room back into the waiting room. I was sobbing, and there was no one to come to my aid; the patients, in their pain, were unaware of me, and the staff keep their distance. At first, I even took the wrong coat. Somehow or other I got out into the street. I felt so wretched, so dizzy. Incapable of thinking about the next step,

I dragged myself to the nearest seat and sat down in the cold winter sunshine.

Now I knew what I had; and it meant, again, that I had to pick myself up and fight. "No, I'm not giving in yet!" Arriving home, where my cats were waiting for me, I picked them both up and nuzzled them; as so often, I was sorry that cats can't talk. From the start, I knew that I would have to go this way alone. First I wanted to find out more about this type of dementia. Next, I resolved to accept my new disabilities and live with them, and – in retrospect, perhaps most difficult of all – not to show what was going on in my innermost self.

My son saw a mother who was a bit different from before, more impatient, exhausted, and with severe variations in her capabilities. I had a good grip on myself, didn't moan, and tried not to burden him with my fears. At the time I considered it important not to upset him. So soon before the school-leaving exam, he needed to be able to concentrate entirely on school. It took some time for me to notice that my son was growing more mature because of my illness, and that the dementia was giving rise to spiritual kinship. How lovely – for we became an indomitable team.

A few days after the diagnosis I decided to read through the leaflet that the doctor had placed in my hand. It was about the Alzheimer's Society, and the various kinds of support for patients and those around them. In principle it was clear to me that I had to have help; but admitting this to myself and others was hugely difficult for me. To say: "Here I am. I am someone who is weak and needs help," wasn't me. I was a "doer". I sat in front of the telephone, as if turned to stone. What was I to say? Perhaps: "Hello, I have dementia. Can you help me?" Fear of saying it, and thereby making the dementia a reality, inhibited me. If I went down that road and openly admitted my illness to others, then what had been my life up to now was over; of that I was convinced. But if it had to be, I would prefer to disclose myself to strangers, and not my friends, acquaintances, neighbours or clients. "What would they think of me? They wouldn't take me seriously any more," flashed through my mind. I could still hear too clearly in my ears the embarrassing "How daft can you be?" as had often happened in the previous few months when I was unable to follow a conversation properly.

Let's be honest – what image do we have of people with dementia? People with dementia are old, in need of care, helpless and dependent. They can't look after themselves or their children, and certainly can't live unsupervised in their own home. They need care, if possible round the clock: because they are always running away, getting lost, are inappropriately dressed, and have simply "lost it". But all of that didn't apply to me. I was neither old, nor unable to look after myself. No, I was still Helga Rohra, eloquent, successful, educated and, of late, perhaps a bit off the wall. But even so, I *was* badly in need of support, because my financial reserves were slowly dwindling. So I pulled myself together and called the Munich Alzheimer's Society.

A very calm, empathic voice answered. Instantly I felt understanding, began to get a sense of "you are not alone". "Shall we come and see you, or would you rather come here?" asked the friendly voice. Ask strangers into my flat? I was too ashamed for that. Because of my inability to move anything from left to right, it was in total chaos. In the flat, it seemed to me, there was an air of depression and fear of the future... "No thanks, I'll come to you," was my brief, and possibly rather curt, reply.

# SEVEN

# About Lewy Body dementia and how it has been for me

When my doctor gave me the diagnosis in January 2009, the word "dementia" was sufficient in itself to fill me with fear and horror. Like many other people, I associated the word with degradation, decline, memory loss, and ultimately the increasing loss of autonomy and independence. In addition to that, the concepts of dementia and Alzheimer's were one and the same. What this special form of dementia would mean for me, I did not yet know. Thinking about that didn't even occur to me at first. Only in the following weeks and months did I get to grips with Lewy Body dementia and learn, for example, how it differs from Alzheimer's dementia.

Lewy Body dementia goes by different names: sometimes in English it is called "dementia with Lewy Bodies" (DLB). As is customary in medicine, I shall use the abbreviation DLB. DLB was first described at the beginning of the twentieth century by a German neurologist, H. Lewy. He found the Lewy bodies that were named after him in certain brain cells of patients with Parkinson's. DLB is closely related to the dementia that can manifest in Parkinson's Disease. However, in DLB the dementia symptoms come first, before the Parkinson's syndrome with its quite specific effects.

I won't bore you here with a medical treatise. If you are interested in detailed medical facts, you will find further reading, on the websites of the Alzheimer's Societies. But I should warn you: think carefully about what information you really need. In particular, if you notice particular symptoms in yourself, don't automatically assume you have a particular type of dementia. Reference books and also websites frequently describe every facet of the symptoms of types of dementia. Whether and when these appear, however, depends on the individual case. Whether any of it applies to you, no one can say for certain. In particular, don't trust statistics, since they are never related to your individual situation. Do you suppose that the average grades of a school class can tell you anything about your child's punctuation mistakes in their last dictation? Therefore you should regard all sources of information with detachment, and a kind of equanimity. Things are not always as bad as they seem. On no account should you analyse yourself or people close to you. Seek advice from either a doctor whom you trust, or an appropriate information centre.

What I am concerned with here is something different. I would like to show you that dementia manifests in different forms, each of which has a distinct course of development and partly specific symptoms. As you may know, dementia is an umbrella term that covers a range of different illnesses that cause similar symptoms. The most common and most familiar form is, without a doubt, Alzheimer's. However, be aware that up to now there has been no precise understanding of what processes in the brain count as causes of Alzheimer's. Second in terms of frequency are the vascular dementias, where changes in cerebral blood flow are a substantial cause of symptoms. In comparison with these two forms of dementia, DLB is rare. Its prevalence is scientifically controversial, but you can take it that ten per cent of people with dementia have DLB.

As with other forms of dementia, a diagnosis of DLB isn't 100 per cent certain. Even with the most advanced imaging techniques, it is impossible to reach an unequivocal diagnosis of DLB. So diagnosis is still done, as before, on the basis of symptoms that partially distinguish DLB from Alzheimer's. Among the characteristics of DLB are progressive memory malfunction, variable levels of mental ability over the course of a day, and distinctive visual hallucinations. Linguistic abilities, on the other hand, are often not impaired until the later stages. Some of the symptoms that are described in the medical literature are ones that I perceive in myself, others not. In particular, I don't have the typical signs of Parkinson's. Of all my symptoms, my visual hallucinations concern me the most intensely, since I had never known anything of the sort prior to having dementia. Other impairments, such as problems with memory and concentration, I was already familiar with, albeit in milder forms than with dementia. I think these are the easiest problems for someone in good health to understand. Everyone must have doubted their memory at some time or other, or experienced difficulty concentrating. Sometimes a late night following a festive occasion is enough to bring on similar symptoms.

Hallucinations, for me, were quite a different story. The first time I had visual hallucinations, at the end of 2008, I was afraid that I was simply going mad. "Now you're cracking up, Helga," I would say to myself, picturing myself in a closed institution. Fortunately things turned out differently. It's difficult to describe my experience of these hallucinations; however, try to imagine that in your field of vision, at a distance of about ten metres, there is a screen on which a silent film is continuously running, and you yourself are playing one of the main parts in it. On this screen I see scenes from my life, constantly changing and with no connnection whatsoever between them. One moment I see myself as a child, having a nappy put on by my mother, and although I have no photos from that time and actually have no way of knowing what I looked like as a baby, I am certain that I am the child on the changing table. The next moment I see my son's confirmation, and then I am somewhere in Israel with my ex-husband, then suddenly at a conference, etc., etc. I'm pleased to say that all the scenes I see are happy ones. That is, I never see horror scenes, which can certainly happen for other people. I have no influence over the content of my silent films, and none over whether there is one or not. However, I *can* choose whether to pay attention to the film or whether to ignore it, in the same way that you can focus on a movement on the rim of your visual field. It's true that my ability to take no notice of the film depends very much on what state I am in on a given day. If I am agitated or exhausted, the hallucination intrudes into the foreground of my perception. You could compare that, up to a point, with your partner snoring: if you are feeling well and are relaxed, then you can fall asleep in spite of the snoring beside you. But if you badly need to rest because you are already exhausted, it's difficult to filter out the disturbance, and the more worked up you get about it, the less you can ignore it, until finally all you are aware of is the snoring, which forces everything else out of your consciousness. That is exactly how it is with my visual hallucinations when I go to bed. Overall, therefore, I suppose I get too little sleep. For a while, on my doctor's recommendation, I tried using sleeping pills, which did help me to fall asleep. However, it was not refreshing sleep, and the next morning I would feel absolutely whacked. Over time I have learnt to calm myself with breathing and relaxation exercises, to the point that I can drop off to sleep fairly well.

One topic that I am constantly asked about is medication, so I would like to deal with it briefly here. The question of whether medications for symptoms of dementia are useful or not, whether the side effects outweigh the benefits or not, is hotly debated by the experts. I cannot, and prefer not to, join in this debate. But I make no secret of the fact that I do use this type of medication. Thanks to the preparation – a medicated plaster that I stick onto my skin every day – I feel more alert and mentally fit. Conversely, when I don't put the plaster on, everything appears stiff and in slow motion. So far I have been spared from side effects, except for some annoying skin irritations. Ultimately everyone has to decide for themselves whether this kind of medication is of benefit or not. Far be it from me to make any general recommendation either for or against drugs.

In addition to this medication, I take an anti-depressant every day, which I find of great benefit. Especially in the early stages of, indeed before the diagnosis was confirmed, I used to suffer from depression, which manifested on the one hand in a deep sadness, such that I would frequently burst into tears for no obvious reason; and on the other hand, I would be paralysed by a leaden lack of motivation. On many days I was incapable of so much as making myself a coffee. My willpower was insufficient for even the slightest of activities. With the help of the anti-depressant, these symptoms have markedly improved.

In retrospect, I am convinced that the depression was amplifying some of the symptoms of dementia to the extreme. I noticed it in my abilities as a linguist. At the end of 2008, and continuing into the first six months of 2009, I was unable to speak English, or even understand it, let alone French. Even my second mother tongue, Romanian, was practically unavailable to me. This improved significantly as the depression diminished. However, I have not regained the ability to translate simultaneously from one language into another. Nevertheless, today I can converse in foreign languages without any problems, and also follow specialist lectures. Of course, this improvement is not solely due to medication. It has a lot to do with the fact that I have learnt to accept dementia as part of my life, and that nowadays my fears for the future, especially financial ones, no longer have such a powerful impact on my thinking. I am not papering over the cracks; some things have got worse with time, my memory leaves me in the lurch more often, my sense of direction has been badly affected, and I am finding it increasingly difficult to ignore the hallucinations. On the other hand, I have developed strategies that enable me to partially mitigate the deficits.

What the future looks like, I don't know. Of course I know the statistics that predict the duration of this illness as seven to eight years; but whether the statistics are right is by no means certain. And anyway, who is helped by knowing statistics like this? How do I know whether my dementia will follow an average course? Leave the numbers games to the experts. I, at any rate, have decided to ignore the statistics. Well, that's not entirely true, since I have in fact resolved to show the statisticians, and live well with my dementia for some decades to come.

# EIGHT

# Summer 2009: At the bottom of the ladder and first aid from the Alzheimer's Society

After I had called the Munich Alzheimer's Society, I set off to go there the very next day, the motivation for this coming at some cost because of my stricken sense of direction. All the same, I had to travel across the city by underground and tram to reach the advice centre. That was my understanding of the abstract sketch in the flyer showing how to get there. Only after I had wandered across the city without success for several hours, and finally rung the Alzheimer's Society again in desperation, did I find out what the route description meant: the advice centre *could not* be reached by either the No. 2 underground line, nor by the No. 19 tram. However, I had assumed that you obviously had to take first the underground and then the tram – hence my involuntary tour of the city.

When I finally reached the advice centre, I was received by a concerned member of the team, Doris Wohlrab, whose great sympathy instantly aroused my trust. Frau Wohlrab, a gerontologist by profession, worked at the Alzheimer's Society as a counsellor for people with dementia and those close to them, and also led various groups and discussion circles.

With her I could talk quite openly about myself, the changes in my life, and my fears. I had confidence in Frau Wohlrab, who listened to me patiently and seemed to know a great deal about the needs and problems of younger people with dementia. Some time afterwards I learned that she is an acknowledged expert in this field, and devotes the greater part of her time to the subject. With her sensitivity to the difficulties people have in dealing openly with their dementia, she was positively predestined for this work.

In the course of our first conversations she asked me to produce my documents, my medical certificate and fixed appointments. I was glad to do so, as I was no longer up to thinking about my responsibilities on my own. We decided between us that I would join a group of patients with dementia straight away. The group was called *TrotzDem*, meaning "Despite Dementia". The group always met early on Monday evenings. I liked the idea of getting to know other patients – people with whom I would be able to talk openly about my problems, who would understand me and know what

I was talking about, because they had probably had the same experiences.

The following Monday I set off in very good time. I already knew from experience that places looked very different and strange to me as soon as the light conditions changed. My son wrote down for me the precise stops where I would need to get on and off – for although Munich is a marvellous city, I had no inclination to do another tour of it. Jens presumably thought that I was volunteering at the Alzheimer's Society, since I was now going regularly to the advice centre. As yet, he knew nothing about my diagnosis. He was only puzzled that I was always so meticulous about getting ready for Monday evenings.

To this day, I still have a vivid pictorial memory of going into the room with the other patients. Elderly ladies and gentlemen were sitting at a long table, a card with their name on it in front of each one. I sat down next to an elderly lady and waited uncertainly to see what I was in for in this group. I watched the others. They were laughing, a few were chatting, there was tea and biscuits. They all appeared quite normal; there was something almost like a regulars' table in a pub about the gathering. Then two facilitators came in. One of the two, Frau Wohlrab, I already knew. We began with a round of introductions in which each person was to say something about themselves. I heard about the others' families, retirement, grown-up children, and grandchildren. During the conversation I was struck by their frailties. Like myself, many didn't answer the question they had been asked, but replied with something entirely different. Many came up with unusual associations, and their words didn't say what they were meant to. It is true that many of the others had symptoms, if their limitations can be termed thus, that were mostly more pronounced than my own – nevertheless, I sensed in the other participants the same helplessness that I was often overcome with myself.

After a while, more people joined our group. As if it were the obvious thing to expect, pairs formed, and only then did I understand the concept of the group. Frau Wohlrab had indeed told me about two parallel groups – but I suppose that in our first conversation I was so preoccupied with myself and my hopes that I hadn't heard her correctly. So two groups were involved, meeting at the same time, in different rooms. The one that I had been taking part in was for the people with dementia. The other group was made up of their relatives, and at the end of the group sessions everyone came together in one room.

Now I discovered that a proportion of the patients and their relatives had been together for years on the path that dementia had laid down for them, that the loved ones felt bound by duty, and the patients grateful. "Oh, my God," I thought to myself. "It can't be like that for you. You're in a completely different situation, your worries are quite different. You don't want to be dependent on anyone!" I sat bolt upright, growing more rigid by the minute. I went home with mixed feelings. Apparently it was like this: patients and their relatives go the same way together. Suffering seemed to bond them with one another, but did it also make them strong?

I attended the group for a few more weeks, even though I felt increasingly that my needs were not being catered for. How I would have liked to be doing something with music, and perhaps relaxation exercises or something creative. Sometimes I would have preferred a more pleasant atmosphere when things got serious – as serious as the word "dementia" sounds. I was looking for something to draw strength from. I felt especially out of place when the two groups came together. What was I doing there, as a single woman looking after herself? Not to mention the impression I occasionally had that the relatives were making the "patient" condition worse. I recall one elderly gentleman who, despite his impairments, seemed open and energetic as long as we were among ourselves – but as soon as his wife came along, going, "Dad, your shirt, Dad, you're sitting all lop-sided again. Dad, would you like some tea?" I could see him literally collapsing. There it was again, the well-meaning advice of those who are fit in mind and know what's good for us. Their caring made them deaf and blind to our desire for autonomy and self-determination. Not that the wife would have patronised her husband deliberately; it was her protective instinct that made her behave that way. Among ourselves, those of us with dementia often exchanged views about it, mostly with a sense of humour: "The ones who are disturbed are actually the relatives," we joked, and were in agreement that the relatives ought to be put into therapy, in the same way they had done with some of the patients. It's always easy to say that sort of thing within a protected group space. Saying it to one's nearest and dearest on whom one may, after all, be dependent, or making it public, is another matter entirely.

Many of the group members had retired long before the first symptoms appeared. With a pension and health insurance, their financial situation was settled; there was no threat to their existence. It is often very different for younger people like me who are wrenched out of professional life and confront an abrupt loss of social status. Although I shared many worries and needs with the older people, my requirements still varied considerably from theirs. I didn't want to hear presentations about the difference between an advance directive and power of attorney. I certainly didn't want to know a range of options for living in old age, or how to find a good care home. That is all still too far off.

The Despite Dementia group is not a self-help group in the full sense of the word, much more a range of psycho-educational seminars. The concept of psycho-education is linked with an approach that is used for many kinds of mental illness, which holds that coming to terms with it is made easier by providing specialist information, and by mutual exchange of experiences in dealing with the illness. Therefore every Despite Dementia group evening came under the heading of a topic to be discussed at the session: "Diagnosis", "Medication", "Power of Attorney" and the like. However, it would be true to say that the "purist" approach is not used in Munich. The planned topics merely provided a certain outline for the session, but the conversation would sometimes develop along completely different lines, depending on what was important to the participants. Mostly, too, Frau Wohlrab did not attempt to guide the conversation back to the topic, but would allow plenty of space for patients' concerns, which I found very accommodating. My need to talk was much too great, as was my desire for mutual exchange and shared activities, for me to be interested in a discussion, and I think the others felt the same.

Most of the Despite Dementia group members had more obvious impairments, and were also mostly substantially older than me. Nevertheless, I always tried to gain something from the group evenings, if only praise for being so strong, and so good at getting to grips with my situation.

After several weeks I asked to talk to Frau Wohlrab, since of late I had been feeling out of place in this group.

She explained that she had recommended this package to me to help me out of my isolation, and enable me to talk to others who were in a similar situation. But she confirmed my impression that over the weeks I had become more composed and was no longer so deep in the dungeon of depression. She suggested, therefore, that I should move to a different group that would be starting shortly. It was called DeMiL – Dementia in the Middle of Life – and was specially for people with dementia under the age of 65. The concept of the groups in tandem applied to this package too: here too, relatives and patients had parallel meetings and came together at the end of sessions. I was happy to accept this fly in the ointment if I had the chance of meeting people of my own age. With hindsight, that was definitely the right decision, for in DeMiL I was to meet people with whom I remain friends to this day.

I myself now started on the pills and plasters that my doctor had prescribed for me. I always told him about the group and my own circumstances. I felt understood by my doctor. Gradually my fighting spirit and courage to face life returned. Nevertheless, my fears for the future, my worries about being able to pay the rent and having the wherewithal to live, still governed my life for the time being. It was the beginning of my battle not only with the symptoms of this uncommon dementia, but also with the wheels of bureaucracy, and ultimately a fight for survival.

# NINE

# Doing battle with the bureaucrats

In April 2009 my financial reserves were pretty much all gone. It had been obvious for months that this was going to happen sooner or later, unless I managed to get back into professional work. But that was unthinkable. Quite apart from my fragmentary foreign vocabulary and my woefully brief attention span, I was preoccupied with striking a balance between dementia and my daily routine. Despite the looming financial catastrophe, pride and shame had so far deterred me from claiming assistance from the state. Only after patient and lengthy persuasion on the part of Frau Wohlrab did I bring myself to make the relevant applications.

Since I had always worked freelance, I had never paid unemployment insurance contributions – something that only employees are entitled to do – so I wasn't able to claim Unemployment Benefit I, but had to apply directly for Unemployment Benefit II, better known as Hartz IV.

After I had worked my way through the relevant forms, I went to my first appointment with the Employment Agency. I deliberately say "worked" here, as these forms are a challenge even for those in a good state of health. With dementia you haven't a chance of managing without assistance, and all I can say is, in order to achieve this task, get support from independent sources. Errors made in filling in the application forms can lead to benefit being calculated incorrectly, or even none at all being awarded. You can, it's true, appeal against the benefit decision, but, from experience, that will delay payment of funds.

While the case worker was still busy with the papers and his PC, his colleague called out to me: "We can make an appointment for the placement interview straight away." So I made an appointment with the young woman for two and a half weeks later, in the hope that by then her colleague would have issued me the money to pay the rent. But it was not to be; the money didn't arrive until June, two months late. If Frau Wohlrab from the Alzheimer's Society hadn't intervened on my behalf, my landlord would have thrown me out of my flat.

On the day appointed I was standing in front of the so-called placement officer. In order to remove all doubt at the beginning, I indicated straight away that I was prepared to accept any work within the scope of my abilities: "Whatever you've got, even if the basic rate is only 400 euros, or, if you like, a one-euro job." I pointed out that I was handicapped, but added: "I'm willing to work for my money." "Well, what's the matter with you?" I answered bravely, without crying: "I don't know how much medical knowledge you have. Do you know what dementia is?" "Yes, yes, you've got Alzheimer's," she said. To which I replied, "No, I haven't got Alzheimer's. I'm not that old. But I do have a form of dementia."

I tell you, she turned pale and then stood up, saying, "I'm just going to see my line manager, I'll have to ask her. I've never had a case like this before," and she left me sitting there like an idiot, and didn't come back. I then asked her colleague what I should do – wait, or go away. He too was at a loss. And so I waited. After an eternity she came back and said, "In your case, this is how it is: you've got to see an assessor. And as far as I can see, you're in a different category. You aren't capable of working for more than three hours a day."

I was stunned, and said, "But even I don't know how much work I can do. Isn't there someone who deals with people like me, with a neurological condition? Haven't you got anything for me?" "No," she replied, "I'm sending you to see the assessor first, there's nothing we can do until then." "And what am I to live on?" "My colleague will issue the money for your rent and the €359 a month Unemployment Benefit II."

TEN

# Appointment
# with the assessor

The case worker at the Employment Agency had said there was nothing she could do for me until I had been to the assessor, and she gave me an appointment for 5 August 2009. On 4 August, however, she sent me a so-called placement proposal for a job that was out of the question for me – and this in spite of the fact that I hadn't even seen the assessor. I thought to myself, the good woman must be demented herself. Anyway, I didn't respond to it.

The appointment with the assessor lasted almost half a day. First, you give your details, and then they are checked. "You've got a disabled person's ID card, severely handicapped by 50 per cent." "Yes," I said, "but that's nothing to do with the dementia. That relates to having cancer in 2003, from which I've now recovered. In the meantime, I've been working." Then followed a painstaking examination of my physical and mental health. At intervals, repeatedly, I asked about the results and whether I was still within the normal range. However, I got no answer, except the rebuke that the assessment would be sent to me by post. At the end of the examination I was asked what I had in mind to do – in answer to which I insisted that I wanted to work, only I didn't yet know what, and for a start I needed to find out what I was capable of. "But I do want to work!"

Naively, I had assumed that at the assessment I would be told what sort of job was still suitable for me, and what kind of support might be helpful for me, and to what extent. But the assessment isn't about that at all: it merely determines whether or not you can work for more than three hours a day – since, if you can't work for three hours a day, you are deemed unemployable and won't get Unemployment Benefit II, but will have to apply for social security. Support options or rehabilitation, such as I was hoping for, are apparently not available. Once, almost two years later, I met a doctor at some event, who also did this kind of assessment. He told me that many people want not a certificate of capacity for work, but the opposite, so that they can apply for a retirement pension. Retirement was far from my thoughts; after all, I was only 55 years old.

Some time later I received the assessment by post, and it said: "Full disability pension recommended" on the basis that I was incapable of working for three hours a day. Soon after that came the decision from the Employment Agency: as I was unable to work for at least three hours a day, I was unemployable. Therefore they were not responsible for me, and would stop my benefit; I might possibly be able to claim social security, which I could apply for c/o Frau Lehmann.[1]

Fair enough; I certainly wouldn't be able to work for three hours a day as an interpreter, not even for three minutes, to be honest. But some sort of easy office work – be it only folding bills and sticking them into envelopes, part-time, as far as I was concerned – was a possibility. But matters of support, identifying resources, or proposals for rehabilitation or reintegration into the labour market, did not come into the assessment procedure, as far as I could see.

Having no alternative, I tried to telephone this Frau Lehmann from Social Security, but either the line was engaged or the answerphone came on. You hope in vain for someone to call you back. It went on like that for a week. Finally I set off for the Munich branch of Social Services, a massive administrative centre that apparently has to be protected from the needy by security people and armed police officers. No chance of getting past the barrier. Frau Lehmann, then, was inaccessible not only by phone but physically as well. By gracious permission of the fierce reception staff, I left a note for Frau Lehmann, asking her to call me.

And Frau Lehmann did indeed materialise in the form of a telephone call: "Frau Rohra, you may be

---

1    Not her real name.

eligible for other payments. But first there is the question of untouchable assets.[2] You have a life insurance policy." She went on to demand that I should first use up this life insurance. Don't misunderstand what I am saying: at the time, my meagre nest egg was worth roughly €3,000.

Of course I had declared this insurance policy. However, there was a snag, and I replied, "Yes, Frau Lehmann, but it's tied up as security." "Can you provide evidence of that?" I said, "Listen, please may I come and see you in the office? I have difficulty explaining things like this over the phone."

Now as then, I feel cornered and as if paralysed if I'm not given time to think and have to get my head round complicated facts at the drop of a hat. Anyway, I added, "Look, I can't recall so quickly, but I believe I've already given all the documentation to your colleague at the Employment Agency." "Very well," she replied, "come along, I'll leave the application forms here." I then went back to Social Services, and once again, as expected, I was not allowed in. Equipped with a few blank forms that could just as well have been sent by post, I left the inhospitable place. I filled in all the forms at home and then handed them in at the Social Security office – with a fresh request for Frau Lehmann to call me, seeing that once again she had not been willing to see me.

---

2    According to German social legislation "untouchable assets" are those in excess of the amount needed to cover the costs of subsistence.

She called on 7 October: "I've found the documentation for the insurance. I'm sorry to tell you that you'll have to use up the €3,000 from the life insurance policy, otherwise you can't get any benefit." I instantly replied that I couldn't use the life insurance policy because it was being used as security. She retorted, "You must understand that we can't support people with assets."

My objection that this was not an asset, and that I was sick and had to take care of my autistic son, was swept aside with the remark, "That's got nothing to do with it. But you can appeal." "Of course I shall appeal, but I can't do it in writing. It does say that you can submit an appeal by getting it recorded by the caseworker. It would help me a great deal if I could do it that way." "No, you've got it wrong" came the answer to that. "'Recording' means that you have to write it down and hand it in."

Once again it was Frau Wohlrab from the Alzheimer's Society who came to the rescue and opened doors for me. On a recent training course she had met a lady from the Specialist Integration Service, an authority whose principal task is integration at work and support for people with disabilities. Although in the meantime my need for a companion on visits to government offices had been covered, we arranged an appointment at the Specialist Integration Service, since otherwise I would have missed the deadline for my appeal.

Just as everywhere else I had been so far, once we had said "Hello" this caseworker too must have asked the following two questions: first, was I actually competent? And second, how was I going to pay the fee for the case? As put to me, it went something like this: "Give me everything you've got – ID, disabled person's pass. Have you got a client number at the Employment Agency? First, I've got to record your details." She disappeared behind a screen with my papers and left me sitting in the corner. Contentedly sipping her coffee, she indulged in an orgy of paper-shuffling and keyboard-clattering. Communication in the form of inquiring about my needs or concerns was apparently not part of the procedure. "Never mind, what matters now is that she's helping me," I thought – but there was no help in sight.

After the bureaucratic prologue, I got to tell my story. I had scarcely finished before she cried, gesticulating wildly, "You must go to the press with this. What an example. I've never heard such a story!" I interrupted her: "The press? I don't want to go to the press. Do you know what I'd like? I'd like you to help me get three hours' work a day somewhere or other. I don't want to retire yet." No inquiry as to what I could or would like to do – just the pithy statement that, "Actually it's very difficult, integration. There isn't anything. We're in an economic crisis; and what do you want it for anyway?" To which I replied, "I feel too young. I still have capabilities, and I want to have a purpose in my life." The reaction was shattering: "Then do voluntary work. It's true that all you'll get is coffee, but there's your purpose." "But I've got to have something to live on. Look, Social Security have told me that I'm not getting anything more." In answer to which: "Well, here's my advice to you. You need a solicitor. One who will represent you in social law." "Aha, social law, you say, and where should I go with that?" "I can't say exactly, but you must go to the Social Court. I'm only responsible for work integration," she said, "and, Frau Rohra – then come and let me know how you got on." She gave me her card and we said goodbye.

That's what they call an "integration specialist". I had gone there in the hope of getting help, but apart from advice to go to the Social Court and tell my story to the press, nothing had come of it. In my frustration I sobbed all the way home and begged: "Dear God, give me strength to muster my thoughts and submit an appeal to Social Security. Otherwise I'm going to be thrown out of my home."

With Frau Wohlrab's support it reached a happy end late in autumn 2009, and positive decisions from Social Security as well as the pension insurance scheme came into effect. Since then I have been receiving a full, reduced earning capacity pension that cannot be revoked, with entitlement to additional earnings of up to €400 a month without forfeit. The pension decision is valid to this day. Up to now I have been neither offered nor allocated any support in looking for opportunities to generate additional income, nor integration assistance intended for people with disabilities. Any chance of that happening? I doubt it!

# ELEVEN

# Autumn and winter 2009: Helen Merlin "Speaking for myself"

In July 2009 two gentlemen who worked for an organisation called Stuttgart Dementia Support visited our DeMiL group, doing research for an article that was to appear in the journal demenz Das Magazin, which they edited. They questioned us group members about, for example, how and when we had noticed the first symptoms, how we came to be diagnosed and what our lives had been like since then. I still remember this interview well, because it was the first time I spoke in public about my dementia. I insisted on remaining anonymous, and I described how I had lost my work because of dementia, and that the Employment Office was not prepared for people like me. It all simply poured out of me: my resentment at the authorities, the feeling of being helplessly exposed to the situation, and also my fear of the future. As I was telling my story I kept bursting into tears, so that by the end of the conversation I was totally exhausted. The two gentlemen then gave each of us a copy of the magazine. I put mine in my bag without looking at it and took it home. It wasn't until several days later that I picked it up, began leafing through it, and in the end read the whole issue from cover to cover. Although many of the articles did not deal with the situation of early onset patients (and it was also about problems in the later phases of dementia), I found the magazine interesting. The journal was aimed at patients as well as carers. It should be possible, I thought, to place equal emphasis on to the special situation of early onset patients. Perhaps by doing that I could also meet other people who, like me, were solitary, in deadlock with the authorities, and felt that they were still capable of meaningful activity.

In October 2009 I was again asked whether I was willing to tell my story. This time it was concerning a book in which exclusively people with dementia were to have their say. I liked the idea. I saw an opportunity to bring my situation before a wider public and speak as the representative of all those who were in a position similar to mine. Certainly, I also had reservations. Would I manage to write a fairly long text, and would I be up to it emotionally? What about my anonymity? Not everyone round about needed to know that I had dementia. As it turned out, these reservations were groundless.

On 22 October 2009 Falko Piest, with assistance from whom I was later to write this book, visited me in Munich to listen to my story. He would take on the writing, I was simply to narrate my story onto tape. In early November I received the transcript from him by email, and was able to make comments and say if I wanted to change anything. It went to and fro in this way a few times until finally my chapter for the book *Speaking for Myself: People with Dementia Have their Say* was ready. Like in the book, I concealed my true identity and published my story under the name of Helen Merlin. It was to be another two months before I gave up the pseudonym.

It was this project that first gave me the idea that this could be a possible sphere of activity in the future. I had worked my way into a new field of expertise – coming to terms with dementia and the challenges it brings with it. With this experience, might there not be a role for me somewhere? Then, in December 2009 I got my first opportunity. The German Alzheimer's Society had issued invitations to an exchange meeting in Kassel for people across the country who were leading groups for early onset patients. Our group leader, Frau Wohlrab, asked which among us would like to go with her. A "colleague" and I immediately volunteered to go to Kassel to represent the patient's viewpoint and give an account of our experiences.

I have no recollection of the individual items on the agenda, but several encounters have remained in my memory – such as the warm welcome from Sylvia Kern, manager of the Alzheimer's Society in Baden-Württemberg, who greeted us by saying she felt honoured and delighted that patients too were participating at the gathering, and thanked us for coming. That touched me deeply. Maybe things like that are being said all the time, but for me those words were something special and it really gave me a boost at the time. There I was, sitting among experts, psychologists and social workers. Once the conference was under way I was able to overcome my inhibitions and make my own contributions to the discussion. Only at lunch did a rather unpleasant situation arise, when two conference delegates insisted on helping me at the buffet. I felt rather overprotected, especially as I hadn't asked for assistance and wasn't out of my depth in the slightest. Nowadays I deal with these infringements with more understanding and good humour. At the time I would feel humiliated if anyone failed to acknowledge my competence.

On 8 January 2010 a journalist from *SPIEGEL* did an interview with members of our DeMiL group, to be published in a special issue on the subject of dementia. By this time I was finding it a lot easier to tell friends about my dementia, but even so, in this article I wanted to appear only as "Helen Merlin". I had no idea that by the time the special issue came out, I would already have given up my pseudonym.

## TWELVE

# Shame, or the problem of being open about symptoms

On the face of it, dementia is nothing to be ashamed of. Anyone can get dementia without deserving it, at a stroke of fate. The symptoms and deficits that are part of the disability are also outside one's personal control. If you're forgetting appointments, places or people, or if you become disorientated all of a sudden, there's nothing you can do about it. Nevertheless, those with the condition often feel guilty when they can no longer function in the way that's familiar to them and others. That's how it was for me, too. Only gradually did I realise that my deficits weren't the result of failure or lack of discipline on my part, but the effects of dementia. The diagnosis helped a great deal in coming to this insight.

When I noticed the first symptoms – forgetfulness, weak concentration, language problems – I said to myself: "Helga, just pull yourself together now!" I had always been very ambitious, worked hard and willingly. I couldn't bear being so incapable, and I put myself under pressure. At the time I had no one with whom to talk openly about my difficulties. My son was about to take his school-leaving exam, and I was certain that he wouldn't pass if I opened up to him.

I didn't want to explain myself to my clients, since that would have been certain to damage my reputation. No one was to find out that the resolute freelance in control of her life had turned into such a wreck.

Of course I could have turned to friends, neighbours and others that I knew. But then Jens might have found out about my troubles from a third party. I wanted to avoid that at all costs. However, what I feared much more than indiscretion was good advice. I was already putting myself under enough pressure; I would certainly not have been able to take any more.

When I finally got the diagnosis of Lewy Body dementia at the beginning of 2009, to begin with "the sky fell in on me", as they say. I was afraid that my limitations would now get even worse – which, by the way, was not in keeping with the facts; but more about that later. On the other hand, the diagnosis also came as a relief. Now I knew that my problems weren't being caused by my lack of discipline, but were the consequences of dementia. The "pull-yourself-together" voice inside my head grew quieter, until in the end it fell silent.

Also, following the diagnosis, I didn't want to spread the word about it straight away. Jens would be busy with his school-leaving exam until June 2009. I continued to leave my friends in the dark as well, and not just for Jens' sake: I would have had no idea how to tell them – just come straight out with "Do you know what, I've got a diagnosis, it's dementia." At the word "dementia" most people immediately think of the alterations of advanced dementia. I didn't want to be linked with those images of helplessness and being looked after. I didn't want to be pitied. I didn't want to hear: "Oh, you poor thing!"

I had overcome so many difficulties in my life already. I felt that pity would have taken away my belief in myself. I am still so young, and I don't even want to think about being looked after. I want to be treated like any normal person of my age. At the time I didn't believe my friends would do that.

# THIRTEEN

# January 2010:
# "THIS MAKES SENSE!" –
# I step out of the shadows

The conference that took place on 28-29 January 2010 was entitled "THIS MAKES SENSE! People with Dementia Get Involved". People with dementia were to talk on the podium about their experiences. Christian Zimmermann from our group had sponsored the event. Richard Taylor from the USA, who had Alzheimer's, was to give a talk, and James McKillop, who also had dementia, had agreed to give a report about his work with the Scottish Dementia Working Group. I was very much looking forward to this event, and so were all the other group members, a number of whom were coming to Stuttgart with their partners. Weeks in advance I was preoccupied with the conference; many of the contributions would be in English. It would definitely be possible to listen to the simultaneous translation through headphones, but I was determined to hear what was said in the original language. I was really excited: "Will I be able to understand the English-speaking visitors? Can I perhaps even talk to them in English?" I hadn't been working as an interpreter for over 18 months; how much was left of my vocabulary?

On entering the conference centre, I felt myself being reminded of old times. How many times had I interpreted at conferences? Collecting the conference folder; pinning my name card onto my suit; the animated conversations of delegates over coffee. The conference began with a song that moved me deeply and instantly created a good atmosphere. Weeks later I heard the song again in a music shop and asked the shop assistant about it. He replied, "Oh, that's ancient. It's 'Walk of Life' by Dire Straits." Never mind how old it was, I bought the CD, and whenever I'm unwell it's wonderful feel-good music.

After Christian Zimmermann, as the sponsor, had opened the conference, one of the next speakers was James McKillop with his report on the work of People with Dementia in Scotland. I was most impressed and said to myself: "We need something like the Scottish Dementia Working Group in Germany too. An organisation of patients, for patients, in which each person contributes whatever they can." What surprised me most was that I could follow James very well, in spite of his Scottish accent. You can't imagine what a boost this gave me: I could still do it, the foreign language was still there, so I wasn't that dotty after all. I did, rather wistfully, glance at the other end of the hall, with the interpreting booths where my colleagues were translating. But I quickly banished a trace of sadness: here I was, sitting in the front row of this conference. On my right sat Dr Peter Whitehouse, a professor and world authority from the USA, who very gallantly paid me a compliment that made me have faith in my personal strengths, and still does today: "Helga, you are doing a great job. You are simply brilliant." He said that after my first public appearance.

How this appearance came about is easily told. On Day Two of the event there was a workshop on the topic of groups for people with dementia. Three group leaders, amongst them our Frau Wohlrab, were to introduce their concepts and describe what was special about their approach. Falko Piest, who was facilitating the workshop, had asked me that morning whether I would like to say something about the benefits of our group from a user's point of view. But as the event was being filmed, it wouldn't make sense to appear under a pseudonym – would I be prepared to abandon the safety of anonymity? Under the influence of the morning's proceedings, and with the awareness that I still had many resources – even my language skills were still fairly good – I agreed; and so I stepped out of the shadows and into the limelight as Helga Rohra.

I received powerful applause for my contribution. Many conference participants came up to me afterwards, congratulated me and encouraged me to continue. From that day on I have been open about my dementia; the Helen Merlin pseudonym no longer has a purpose. The book containing my article was presented at the conference, and I rather regretted having to explain that "Helen Merlin is me." At the time when I had written it I had been unable to imagine that I would ever stand up on a public platform and talk about my experiences of dementia. In the past few months, then, some huge changes had been taking place in my life.

I have never regretted "coming out". On the contrary: since then I have been fundamentally freer in the way I live my life. My game of hide-and-seek had cost me an incredible amount of energy. Following this experience I was at last able to tell everything to my son, who had not been with me in Stuttgart. He took it better than I had expected.

My public appearance at "THIS MAKES SENSE!" was a turning point for me: if, for a few months, I had vaguely toyed with the idea of devoting myself to the cause of those of us with dementia, now I wanted to make a positive effort to promote our best interests. That very day I spoke to Frau Wohlrab, who had accompanied our DeMiL group from Munich, and asked what opportunities she saw for me. She drew my attention to the upcoming elections to the board of the Munich Alzheimer's Society, which were to take place in March: I could stand for election, she said. At first I thought it was a joke. But she was perfectly serious, because she had no doubts about my aptitude for the post. "Well, why not, in fact?" I said to myself, and the same evening told the then chairwoman of the Alzheimer's Society, who was also attending the congress, of my plans. It was in high spirits that our group, and myself especially, celebrated at the hotel bar that evening, late into the night, or the small hours. This indeed was the dawn of a period of my life that I would have considered unimaginable only a short while before.

# FOURTEEN

# March 2010: Thessaloniki – On my own

At the Stuttgart conference there were many experts, journalists, and officials too, who took notice of me. So it came about that the German Alzheimer's Society asked me whether I would like to go to the Alzheimer's Disease International (ADI) Congress in Thessaloniki in Greece. At first I was sceptical, but after reading in the programme that people with the condition would be coming from other countries as well, I plucked up the courage. To begin with, there was a degree of uncertainty regarding the practicalities of taking part. The Alzheimer's Society had indicated that they would be responsible for the costs of travel and accommodation; I should send them the documentation afterwards. But if, like me, you are reliant on social security, the outlay of a few hundred euros for the flight and a hotel instantly makes an enormous hole in your household budget. However, in the short time left there was obviously no chance of arranging a hotel for me. After some beating about the bush I decided to bite the bullet and asked Jens to book me into a cheap hotel. The flight was booked for me by ADI. I was sent a form by email, which I was to print, fill in, sign, scan and return by email. I can write a simple email; I can't attach a file, let alone fill in and scan a form. ADI simply assumed, in the same way as many other organisations, that we will have a "carer" who does things like that for us. I would prefer it if this kind of procedure were easier to deal with. Jens is glad to assist me, no question about that, but all the same I feel disadvantaged in such situations. This applies not only to me. Nowadays familiarity with a PC and Internet access are tacitly taken for granted. Anyone without these has got a problem – with or without dementia. It seems to me that here, too, it's incumbent on the Alzheimer's associations to demolish the barriers – even within their own organisations.

A few days before leaving for Greece I began to keep a diary of my experiences as a "dementia activist". Here's a short excerpt from it:

### 8 March 2010 – Evening before leaving for Thessaloniki

*The few days prior to departure were exciting. I was amazed at my own daring – alone to Munich Airport – check-in – arrival – find hotel. The matter of orientation was what concerned me most. But joyful anticipation of meeting other people with dementia – being present at key discussions/ meetings at the Congress – was more powerful. And I wanted to know for myself: what can you do on your own – without assistance? – A challenge for me, for my memory.*

*Meeting the "Alzheimer's Family" – my group – in the evening before I left was good. Again, that sense of belonging. Such warmth came across as we said goodbye, and again I knew: these people are giving me the strength to fight. I'm speaking up for all of us. I told them about my urge to engage politically – how I came to identify with my name. I felt that it was doing me good to commit myself again – and feeling really excited, I tried to rest for a few hours.*

## 9 March 2010 – Day 1

*An hour before departure from the flat, my friend told me she wouldn't be able to come with me to the airport after all. No need to panic, I thought. Despite dementia, you'll find everything You must give yourself plenty of time, keep calm. So I started hours in advance. I'd booked my ticket online, and the passenger is also expected to check in on their own. That, of course, was more than I could do, and bravely I approached the desk. I asked for help and was treated very kindly by the staff. I set off with my boarding card in the direction of the departure gate. As no one asked to see my passport, I searched rather uncertainly for my gate. It was a case of following one lot of arrows after another. For a time I was walking in circles, but in the end I saw the waiting area for the Thessaloniki flight. Now I still had an hour in hand, so I went all the way back through the jungle of arrows to get myself a cup of coffee. I was going to have a classy start. I was enjoying it, and was sitting punctually in the lounge ready for departure. Then came the mass movement towards the bus that took us to the gangway. I was calm and relaxed. Caught scraps of conversation about the conference. Probably doctors, pharmarceutical company reps. I listened too, waiting for the moment to make a graceful entry into the conversation. Soon it came. Since, unfortunately, I didn't belong to the medical circle, I was branded as being out of my depth for the conference. This professional group's ignorance, and request to find a carer for me, was beyond tasteless. In spite of this, I hoped that on arrival at Thessaloniki Airport they would offer me a place in their taxi to the city centre.*

*There is still a long way to go in educating people about dementia – first, those treating us need to be sensitised to our needs; and then the man in the street.*

*They did not offer me a place in the cab. On arrival at Thessaloniki Airport, first I went with my suitcase to Lost and Found. There I felt safe, and so it proved. The kind lady wrote down all the information I needed to get to my hotel by bus. I got my €0.50 ticket by myself. Soon I discovered that the street names were written only in Greek. Where am I, now? A young man, eye contact. He must speak English – a direct hit! He even squeezed through the crowd to the driver and back to give me the exact details.*

*No sooner said than done. Now I had to walk for a few metres further. No street names in Roman script, and no house numbers. Well, what an adventure. But it was light, and as long as I could ask... In spite of the detour for herself, a lady took me to right to the hotel. Now the check-in. I was given two chip cards and three remote controls.*

*It began with me being unable to open my door. But the maid was hovering around and unlocked it for me. It was pitch black inside. One card was supposed to switch on the electricity. But where? I had to laugh – I fetched the girl back and got her to explain everything, including the remote controls. It was well worth the euro tip I gave her.*

*Unpack quickly, and out into the chill winter sun: it's 4° C.*

*I want to get to the congress building. I have a map in my hand. It's straight ahead – about six kilometers, it's true, and the map was printed in a time before all these building sites, barriers and diversions existed. Now you have to make big detours. After walking for five hours I'm so exhausted that I can't hunt for the congress building any more. No bus comes, either. I need energy and would like something to eat. But there are only street hawkers and clothes markets. Where are the cafés and tavernas?*

*It's getting dark and I have to find my way. The same way back, only on the other side of the road, and there it is; no, I've never been in this street before. I walk even faster, perhaps I'll recognise something. I even walk past my hotel. And once it's completely dark and the street is thronged with people, I can't find anything any more. I'm walking – but inside I'm feeling quite churned up. My eye falls on an illuminated shop window – white as a sheet!*

*Now I absolutely have to sit down. I go into a bodega – just Greeks, having a drink. I get myself a beer and there's a sandwich too – which I eat immediately. A gulp of beer and out into the street with fresh confidence – I ask – I'm taken to the hotel. And I'm amazed how sensitive the little man is. It's the humanity, the human kindness. You either have it, or you don't – and the Greeks have it. I'm writing these lines before I go to sleep. I need to do this, and I'm thankful and proud of myself! Tomorrow, Wednesday 10 March – take-off!*

On the morning of the first day of the conference I got up in a state of anxiety, since stupidly, in spite of my long excursion on the day of arrival, I still didn't know how to get to the Congress Centre. In a situation like this, the thing is to be be open about it and not feel ashamed. In the breakfast room at the hotel I could see some people who I assumed were also going to be at the conference. So I spoke to them in English: "Are you here for the ADI conference?" – "Oh, yes," replied a very nice doctor from India. Straight away we began chatting about the topics on the agenda. At some point he asked what my occupation was, and whether I too was a doctor. I answered that I would feel very flattered if he took me for a doctor, but I was not: "But no, I'm someone who has dementia." To begin with he wouldn't believe me, and thought I was making fun of him. Until I told him more about myself, he was unconvinced. Then we took the bus to the conference centre together, and the same on the following days.

In March 2011 I saw Dr Jacob Roy again at the ADI Conference in Toronto, when he was elected Chair of ADI. He remembered me immediately and we had a nice chat.

I found the conference in Thessaloniki extremely interesting. I couldn't follow the content of all the presentations, it's true, but I tried to grasp as much as I possibly could – if only to keep up my English. What touched me most was meeting the other people with dementia. The organiser had arranged an extra room where we gathered. For each country a representative had been invited, along with a companion – their partner, for the most part. To begin with I felt a bit lost, since I was the only one from Germany, and had come unaccompanied. But the reception, which I shall never forget, was very warm-hearted and open. Hearing about the situation in other countries, what initiatives had been started there, made me rather envious too. As far as patient participation is concerned, Germany is a developing country when compared to many others. Unlike England, for example, where someone like the well-known fantasy author Terry Pratchett has been talking openly about his dementia for years, in Germany there are no public figures who disclose their dementia and speak as ambassadors for us. In Germany we could do with a lot more people with dementia presenting themselves as such. Only this can alter the generally held picture of dementia.

Following the encounter with my "brothers and sisters", as we called ourselves in Thessaloniki, I went back to Germany with a strong sense of motivation. It had to be possible to educate the public better about us folk with dementia. Perhaps I was too highly motivated – at any rate, since getting home I've been using the shoulder bag that each participant received as a handbag. On the bag it says in large lettering: "25th International Conference of Alzheimer's Disease International", with the subtitle "Dementia: Making a Difference".

A few days after the conference I was sitting with this bag in the Underground in Munich; opposite me were two middle-aged ladies. They read the inscription and were so-o-o-o-o shocked that I was promoting the Alzheimer's Society. On my asking what they found shocking about it, or whether it might not rather be that their fear of the idea was causing them discomfort, the prompt reply came: "I thought they were people who can do nothing any more. Who need to be cared for." To which I answered, "Not everyone – there are others too. Would you like to know more?" At once the lady protested: "No, I don't want to think about it. One day it might be me." "Well, maybe it already is you." The two women moved away in silence. "Dementia: Making a Difference". I stand by the difference, and I want to make people see that there is an enormous difference between us folk with dementia and the image that most people have of us. The two ladies' attitude made me sad and furious at the same time. "Now, more than ever," I said to myself.

# FIFTEEN

# My everyday life and how I cope with it

Dementia keeps me constantly on my toes, and no two days are the same. On good days it stays nicely in the background, lets me do what I want, and only moderately hinders me. On bad days it pushes itself forcefully into the foreground and puts obstacles in my way wherever it can. Even in the course of a day, the degree to which I notice it will vary. After getting up, and throughout the morning, I am very aware of it. Everything feels tough, and I make a terrible hash of even the simplest things: I'm in the kitchen and want to make myself a coffee, I'm holding the filter bag in my hand, and it takes me a very long time to remember where I have to put it. And so it goes on until about midday. After that I'm fit until late in the afternoon, when I hit a low point and get so tired that sometimes I have to lie down. After a nap I'm back on the job until shortly after 20.00. This is annoying, of course, as I like to watch a crime drama on television – but after the first half hour I've mostly forgotten what happened at the beginning. To begin with, that scared me a bit, because I would think: "Now you're advanced, the early stage of dementia must be over." Today, I know that these fluctuations during the course of the day are quite normal in Lewy Body dementia, and they no longer frighten me so much. If I'm watching a crime movie with my son, I always get a summary of the past half hour from him, and so I can follow the plot pretty well. Unless I nod off now and then. But you, too, must be familiar with the "TV snooze" phenomenon.

After that I'm at peak fitness again until 2.00 or 3.00 in the morning. That's actually the time when I can concentrate best, and I like to use it to read, or plan the next few days, or write little notes. It is at night, in the dark, when everything is a bit quieter and daytime distractions aren't disturbing me, that dementia leaves me in peace for a while.

For me, set routines are extremely important, and if I can plot my tasks along my daily performance curve, everything goes smoothly enough. The last thing I need is appointments in the morning. I even turn off my telephone in the morning, to avoid being disturbed. For morning appointments I have to make meticulous preparations and put everything out ready the night before, from clothes to whatever documentation I may have to take with me. Otherwise I just wouldn't get it together in the morning. But, regrettably, the world doesn't much run according to my internal clock.

Through coming to terms with my dementia I have learnt to be patient with myself. Of course, that took some time, but today I am more careful in the way I use my abilities and allow myself time, and above all I no longer panic if something unforeseen occurs. You may recall the episode in which I got lost in my own cellar and almost died of fright. It still happens today that I get disorientated and don't know where I am, particularly, if I'm preoccupied or bothered with something – appointments with the authorities, for example. As I'm dependent on financial assistance, I have to go regularly to social services, perhaps to state whether there has been any change in my income situation. Which is a farce, actually. What change would there be? Nevertheless, every time I'm hounded by the fear that my benefit might be reduced, the money for the rent not paid in time, and the like. Thoughts like these distract me, upset my routines, and it may happen that I get the underground lines all mixed up and am suddenly travelling in the wrong direction. Stupidly, I don't spot this straight away, being occupied with other thoughts, and several minutes have passed by the time I notice: "You don't know the names of these stations. How did you get here? Wherever are you?" At one time, that would send me into a panic. Nowadays I get off at the next stop, take the escalator up to street level, and look for a café. There I sit down, have a coffee and blank out everything around me. Immediately I notice myself calming down. After perhaps half an hour I'm once more capable of action, and then I look for someone I can speak to and ask for help. With time you develop an eye for people who are willing to help and those it's better to avoid, and to tell the truth I have seldom been disappointed. If need be, I could call my son and ask him to fetch me. Fortunately I haven't yet had to use this option, but this lifeline gives me a sense of security nevertheless.

I never leave home without my mobile, and mostly agree with Jens what time I will be back. If it gets later, he calls me and gallantly asks whether I've been delayed. So I don't feel I'm being supervised, but I know that someone is looking out for me. A good friend of mine is always very concerned if I have to get to certain appointments, because she knows what my sense of direction is like. She is almost over-solicitous and always wants to know precisely where I will be and when, what I'm doing, whether I've got everything with me. I've explained to her a number of times that while I really appreciate her concern, she is hemming me in, keeping tabs on me and treating me rather like a small child with her efforts. Even so, she doesn't always manage to overcome her attitude. Let's see whether in future we can find a way of easing her anxiety and allowing me to have my freedom.

# 16 March 2010:
# I am elected to the board of the Munich Alzheimer's Society

The Munich Alzheimer's Society originated from a relatives' self-help group in 1986. As the first regional Alzheimer's Society, it was the pioneer in a success story: the founding of over 100 similar societies, under pressure from which the care system was significantly improved. All Alzheimer's Societies pursue the goal of changing the lives of people with dementia and their families for the better, by providing information about dementia and offering various kinds of advice and help. All Alzheimer's Societies stand up for people with dementia by lobbying and providing a point of contact with the political world. But in practically none of these associations are people with dementia members of the relevant decision-making bodies, let alone holders of official positions.

Many of the Societies can be traced back to the initiative of family members and/or experts from the medical and psychosocial professions. Not a few are, as in Munich, the institutionalised extension of a relatives' self-help group. I think there is good reason to assume that the patients whose relatives founded the first societies in the 1980s and 1990s were struggling with the advanced stages of dementia at the time. If only for that reason, they were not involved in either founding or building up the societies. Early diagnosis of dementia has developed in recent decades; prior to that, in the majority of cases, early dementia was presumably mistaken for depression or other forms of mental illness – which, as I experienced at first hand, is still more the rule than the exception today. Younger people with dementia are, therefore, only gradually coming into society's focus, and here the Alzheimer's Societies are no exception.

I have already described how difficult it is, and how difficult it is made, for those of us people with dementia to be open about our disability, even with those we trust the most. Most of us would therefore not wish, or be able, to engage with an interest group. This challenges society as a whole to open up. There need to be – not as the exception, but always and by obligation – forms of participation and governance that allow us to join in discussion and decision making. The motto of the Scottish Dementia Working Group, "Nothing about us, without us", should become the defining principle in Germany as well. This applies particularly to the Alzheimer's Societies.

Obviously this kind of thing is easier said than done. Prejudices have to be dismantled, barriers overcome, and issues about rights clarified. At the end of February, when I announced to the administrator of the Munich Alzheimer's Society that I wanted to stand as a candidate for the Board, the question arose, first, as to what was the legal position was, and whether patients could actually be on the board of an association. Fortunately the issue was resolved with the help of a lawyer:[3] in German company law, legal capacity is a precondition for holding an executive position – but strictly speaking, this applies only to Board members who are representing the association externally, as set out in the articles of association in accordance with the German Civil Code. Someone who counts as belonging to an extended executive Board is not unequivocally bound to have legal capacity. There is, then, considerable scope when drafting a constitution, if an association wishes its Board to be open to people with limited legal capacity. Particularly important is the fact that lack of legal capacity is determined not, as a rule, with reference to the future, but retrospectively. Accordingly, a diagnosis

---

3    See Klie, Thoma (2010) "Fit genug für den Vorstand?: Rechtlich ist mehr möglich als man denkt." ["Fit enough for the Board? More is legally possible than you think."] *dementia-DAS MAGAZIN*, 4, p.36.

of dementia imposes no restriction either on accepting people in the first stage of dementia as members of an association, or on their assuming official positions. Thus the path was open to me as a person whose legal capacity was not in question, either at that time or today. I could stand for election on 16 March 2010.

Along with the invitations to the general meeting the administrator kindly included notice of my intention to stand for election, together with a brief portrait of me, so that the members were prepared. When at last the general meeting was opened, I had difficulty concentrating on the agenda, being in such a state of excitement about the election. Would they vote for me? Was the time ripe for having a patient on the Board? In the preceding days I had received much support. Encouraging words came from my DeMiL group: "Of course we'll vote for you. Why ever not? Just imagine how the Munich Alzheimer's Society would look if they didn't vote for you."

All that might well be, but how would I react if I failed to be elected? Would I blame it on myself, or on dementia? It would be easier to live with a wounded ego, but if I were reduced to my deficits it would be a bitter pill. The agenda item "Election of Board members" came at last. Individuals were to be confirmed in their posts or elected for the first time by acclamation. To my great joy the vote for me was unanimous.

Working on the Board – once the initial insecurities have been overcome – is trouble-free and refreshingly unspectacular. I assume that my colleagues had to learn how to get on with me, and what abilities I was able to bring to the work. Meanwhile, like the other Board members, I join in discussions and take on tasks that arise, as far as my abilities permit. At no time have I felt that I'm a second-rate colleague. Quite the opposite: I am a full, normal member of the team. Do all my colleagues take the same view? I hope so, and at a suitable opportunity, I'll ask them.

# SEVENTEEN

# Spring 2010:
# The media

My election to the board of the Munich Alzheimer's Society caused quite a stir in the media. Three days later the German Alzheimer's Society announced on its web page: "Woman with dementia elected to the Board of an Alzheimer's Society for the first time". The *Süddeutsche Zeitung* must also have caught a whiff of sensation – at any rate, it sent a reporter to the Munich Alzheimer's Society for an interview with me, and a photographer came along too. The interview took up almost half a morning, since I had a lot of explaining to do – for example, that I have Lewy Body dementia and not Alzheimer's, what the difference is between them, and suchlike. The journalist was very interested, listened attentively and asked intelligent questions. Following the interview there was a photography session. The photographer had his own ideas: "Sit by the window. Then I'll take a few pictures of you." However, I didn't like this idea. People have seen loads of pictures of seated, passive patients. "No, I want something dynamic, something with power. The photo ought to be encouraging for people." It was to be a picture of me standing, preferably next to a Munich Alzheimer's Society poster. However, the poster was much higher than I am, and I looked rather lost in front of it. The solution consisted of an adventurous construction made out of two boxes, on top of which I had to climb, to everyone's amusement, supported by member of the Munich Alzheimer's Society team. In the end the photo for the article "I've got dementia – so what?" was accomplished: Helga Rohra, eye-to-eye with the Munich Alzheimer's Society.

The media response to the article in the *Süddeutsche Zeitung* was prompt in coming, and further inquiries for interviews, and invitations to radio broadcasts and TV shows, followed. The media sent their inquiries direct to the Munich Alzheimer's Society; the journalists didn't know my private address and email address, and that was a good thing. In the early days the Munich Alzheimer's Society team would select the inquiries, showing me only the ones they thought were suitable. They did that with the best of intentions, and in order to protect my privacy. Above all they were afraid that I would take on too much – a worry that was certainly not unfounded, in view of the large number of inquiries. Today I can understand the dilemma confronting the social pedagogues. On the one hand they were pleased about my success and knew what a boost it was for me; on the other hand they were afraid of my overdoing things, and of the pit I might fall into once the initial razzmatazz was over.

The fine line that professionals and families of us people with dementia have to tread, between support and development on the one hand, and care and protection on the other, seems to me characteristic of the way people interact with us. All the more important, therefore, are openness and honesty. That applies on both sides, to people with dementia as well as those supporting us. We should also take a good look at ourselves and say what we really need, and where we really are. We can't expect others to divine our requirements. This does presuppose an atmosphere, or better, a climate in which we can express our need for support without fear of being discredited. In my opinion, a first step in this direction is to put an end to society's clichés about people with dementia, and through my public appearances I would like to make a small contribution to this.

Since March 2010 I have answered questions in the press in over two dozen interviews. I have been in various radio and TV talk shows, and have given many talks at events and conferences. My message is always the same: "Don't just look at our disabilities; look for our capabilities. Often we can do much more than you think is possible, no matter how advanced the dementia.

Don't allow us to become isolated and pushed into the margins of society. We want to stay part of it!"

Probably the fact that the media are so interested in me is owing to my largely unimpaired linguistic abilities. "Oh, a lady with dementia who can talk, in several languages, too. Maybe her English is even better than mine," I sometimes seem able to read in people's faces. I don't fit the stereotype and often give the impression of having virtually no impairment, of being a special case, an exceptional phenomenon. But the impression is misleading. There must be tens of thousands of early onset patients able to talk as well as I can – only they are not visible, for whatever reason. The life situations of us with early onset dementia are mostly different from those of people in the advanced stages, and consequently our needs also differ in many respects. Similarly, those supporting us are faced with different demands. But this is precisely what it's all about. Dementia is a spectrum; each case, and the course it takes, is different. Even if the medical models make out the opposite, ultimately they are little more than a statistical net through which an individual case will always fall. However, arguing with them is impossible.

In February 2011 I was invited onto a TV talk show. The title: "The Horror of Dementia". Inappropiate, you would think, as I did; but in spite of it I went, if only to object to the horror scenario and draw attention to the interests of early onset patients. Except that it was probably in vain. There I sat, the only patient among several family carers and a professor of neurology. It was predictable that the discussion would soon focus on the difficult and regrettable situation of relatives with family members with advanced dementia, and so it was: the relatives talked about their pain, described the long drawn-out farewell to a loved one, and told heartbreaking stories from their everyday lives. The facilitator was evidently keen to evoke the "Horror of Dementia" with all available means. Fortunately the guests on the show were still able to keep interposing some positive experiences with people with dementia. But in the end the discussion focused on the end of life.

It will probably be some time before the media do justice to the many facets of dementia and are able, in addition, to encompass the abilities of people with dementia. Until then it's a question of endurance and perseverance. I shall continue to seek publicity where possible. Perhaps in this way I can give others the courage to open up. I'm certain that there are many others out there who can stand up for our cause like me, in public too. Perhaps some day there will be so many of us that we can no longer be ignored. So many that we can organise ourselves and demand loud and clear: "Nothing about us, without us."

# EIGHTEEN

# Speaker at a congress on dementia: "Why many people I speak to declare that I am well"

The night before the Dementia Fair congress on 22 April 2010, I slept particularly badly. My optical hallucination – my film, as I sometimes call it – kept forcing itself into the foreground. It was difficult for me to ignore it, to separate dream from reality. My brain plays this perfidious trick on me mostly in situations when I least need it. For example, when I'm in desperate need of sleep because the next day threatens to be strenuous. You're sure to be familiar with this from your own experience: the night before a big event you go to bed early and can't sleep for excitement. For hour after hour you're tossing and turning and thinking: "Well, if I don't get to sleep soon...I've got to leave at six, I'll have had less than six hours' sleep." Soon it's less than five, then four, then three, and sleep just refuses to come.

What was keeping me awake that night was the prospect of standing up on stage the following day at a dementia congress in Nuremberg. A new dimension was opening up for me. It was just three months since my first public appearance at the "THIS MAKES SENSE!" conference, and here I was, again, going to speak to a hall full of people with a special interest in the phenomenon of dementia: specialists in medicine, social work and caring. Peter Wissmann, one of the sponsors of "THIS MAKES SENSE!", had asked me if I'd like to talk about the impressions and experiences I'd had since going public about my dementia.

To start with I was sceptical as to whether I should accept the invitation: at the time I didn't yet believe that I was up to giving a 45-minute talk. The fear that my memory might leave me in the lurch and withhold the words I needed was too great. In any case, I wanted to spare myself the embarrassment of losing the plot in public. Fortunately, though, we agreed in the preliminary chats that our contribution was to be not so much a lecture as a converstion in public about my experiences. This I could agree to. I would be happy to trust in the rhythm of question-and-answer. All the same, of course, I wanted to prepare for the event and formulate a few thoughts and ideas for myself beforehand. As so often in previous months, I leafed through the chapter in the other book[4] that I had published under the pseudonym

---

4    *Speaking for Myself: People with Dementia Have their Say.*

of "Helen Merlin". Those texts had come into being a good eight months before. Had my stance altered since then, especially since I had been acknowledging my dementia in public? What had been my experiences with that? Apart from a few strange situations, I've had nothing but positive experiences, once I'm open about my handicap. So what was there to go wrong at the congress in Nuremberg?

Thanks to Jens' meticulous planning and his detailed personal itinerary for me, getting to Nuremberg on my own by Intercity train was practically child's play. On the train I looked out for people who were possibly also going to the congress and whom I could tag along with, unfortunately without success. Because of my poor sense of direction I'm naturally happiest simply going along with someone else. But not until I was on the tram from the station to the Exhibition Centre did I get chatting to a lady who, like me, was going to the congress. She was going to run a workshop there on the following day, giving an account of experience she had gained on a placement at a New York care home. This interested me because it would be in English, for a start. We talked all the time we were on the tram, we discussed our experiences in the USA, and I was feeling good. I was a conference delegate among others, was accepted and could hold my own in conversation. Shortly before we got off the tram, however, I felt the need to tell her that I was a person with dementia.

Her first reaction was: "Oh, come on, I don't believe you." "But I am," I replied, "believe me." Followed by her mistrustful gaze, I walked away from the tram stop and towards the Exhibition Centre. In the entrance hall I must have looked a bit lost, since she kindly and discreetly escorted me to the registration area, where we finally parted company. In the end she probably did believe me.

I adapted well to appearing at the congress. We stood on stage and chatted about my experiences. Peter Wissmann introduced me to the audience as a dementia expert, which flattered me, of course, and so we began our conversation. After a while the audience had a chance to ask questions. Some listeners spoke up, introducing themselves by name and giving the names of the organisations they worked for. They asked me the questions that I am always asked. People are interested, for example, in how I noticed that there was something the matter with me. What were the first symptoms and what did it feel like? Where do I get the strength to go on; how do I cope with my life in this society? In the meantime the answers come almost automatically – all I need do is talk about events in my life. The tone was set by a friendly, interested exchange and an attitude of mutual respect – until suddenly, on the right side of the auditorium, a smart, middle-aged gentleman leaned forward to draw attention to himself. The microphone was passed to him and at once he jumped up: "You can't tell me that you're a patient. I've never known someone with dementia to be so articulate," he said.

This frontal attack hit home. My voice literally failed. I had to hang onto the microphone with both hands for fear that my shaking knees would also let me down. If I had given in to my initial impulse, I would have burst into tears in front of all and sundry. My diagnosis was now over a year behind me, and every day I experienced the limitations that dementia imposed on me; I couldn't go on with my profession; I was reliant on Unemployment Benefit. What was this man thinking of, what right did he have to make such an allegation? After a few moments I had collected myself enough to be able to answer back. Peter Wissmann stood next to me the whole time with a concerned look, and was visibly uncertain whether to take the situation in hand, or whether I was strong enough to tackle this presumptuous man.

"My dear sir," I began ironically, "I don't know who you are and I don't know in what capacity you are speaking, but I'm pleased to tell you that there are various forms of dementia, which manifest in different ways. I am not here to justify myself. My diagnosis is far too serious for me to be making anything up here." Delivered in a trembling voice, this was my answer. When I looked around the audience I could feel the warmth and approval of the other delegates, most of whom were likewise irritated by this man's insensitivity.

Drawing strength from their silent approval, I replied to the man, who was about to launch another question: "No, sir, I won't take any more questions from you." In response I received heartfelt applause from the audience. Nevertheless, I was so shattered that I couldn't go on. With tears in my eyes I withdrew to the back of the stage.

Only later did I discover that the gentleman whose accusation had wounded me so badly was a neurologist or psychiatrist from Frankfurt. To this day I cannot comprehend his insinuation. Why would anyone think of making a false claim to have dementia?

Although there has been no repetition of such an allegation so far, I do occasionally sense, in quite a few people I talk to, a degree of doubt regarding my diagnosis. This may be due to the fact that the impairments in my linguistic abilities are small, especially as my difficulties with word-finding have significantly improved since I've largely recovered from my initial depression. Working with languages determined my entire professional life, so I attribute the stability of my capacity for language to my sizeable reserves in this domain. Whether this supposition stands up to scientific scrutiny is, of course, not for me to say, and it is not, in fact, important to me. The fact is that I can cover up my other limitations caused by dementia with inconsequential chat. To this extent I may not come across as a typical dementia patient.

But do they even exist – typical people with dementia? Or isn't it rather our representation of how a typical person with dementia ought to be, shaped by our own fears and by images of the changes that advanced dementia brings? I'm repeating myself when I say that dementia is always envisaged from the end point, and that in our imagination people with dementia are (must be) old, disorientated and helpless. I can find no other explanation for the tacit or openly expressed doubts as to my diagnosis that I occasionally encounter.

I keep reading or hearing the number 1.2 million. This is the estimated number of people with dementia in Germany – and I say "estimated" deliberately, since the basis for this figure is ultimately an extrapolation from separate, limited surveys of the population as a whole. There are no exact figures – for one thing, because no centralised register for dementia exists in Germany, such as does exist for cancer, for example; for another, as I personally discovered, dementias are difficult to diagnose. But let's suppose that 1.2 million is correct. Then it would encompass the full range of severity of forms of the disease, from mild to very severe. Now, we can all see at a glance that the majority of people with dementia are not suffering from an advanced stage of the disease, since this estimated 1.2 million cannot be exclusively people in need of constant care. No, the vast majority of those affected are living among us more or less inconspicuously. Many of them probably don't yet even know that they have dementia, and link the symptoms with other problems – just as I did, to begin with. What I mean to say, is that dementia is for the most part invisible in the public domain. Our disability doesn't meet the eye; only our behaviour might appear odd, if you look more closely and if, as in my case, you can't instantly tell by listening to us, there's a certain disparity between stereotype and reality. Nevertheless, I would not have expected a medical specialist to have such a narrow view of dementia, and above all, of people with dementia. Possibly, in his practice, that doctor had met predominantly people with profound impairments. Possibly my age tripped him up; such early onset is pretty rare. In the final analysis, that's exactly what he said: he had never met anyone like me. But concluding from that that a case like mine could not exist is simply arrogant and unprofessional.

# NINETEEN

# July 2010:
# At the golf course

For over two years I've been taking more or less regular advantage of the special groups run by the Alzheimer's Society for people with dementia, and I remain convinced of the effectiveness of these groups – although the importance of the group in my life has shifted with time. This shift is connected, I think, with my needs in respect of the contents of the group, or its thematic focus. The first time I went to a group, directly following my diagnosis, I wanted to find out more about dementia in general. I was hoping to learn from other patients about how they coped, what tips and tricks they had worked out for themselves that could be helpful for me in dealing with everyday problems. Presumably it was the same for the other group members, as the conversations focused on this area. What effect does dementia have on your family or partner? How do I find my way around my neighbourhood? What medical or therapeutic possibilities are available to us? These were the most frequently discussed questions.

As time went on, our interests changed. The questions around dementia slipped into the background and other topics gained in importance. In many group members, as in me too, one sensed the desire for a "normal" life. With the group's help we had managed to integrate dementia reasonably well into our lives and daily activities, and we were yearning for the next step. We wanted, just like all human beings, to participate in social life, culture or sport. What we had in mind here were not activities such as the ones proposed by experts as being particularly suitable for people with dementia – I'm referring to choices like memory training or reminiscence. Don't get me wrong, I'm not rejecting this kind of thing outright. In certain situations activities to improve mental ability are appropriate and desired by patients. However, they tend to focus on the participants' impairments and promise to improve or overcome specific cognitive limitations. We, on the other hand, were hoping for activities that did justice to our abilities and resources. That is, we wanted to do things that "normal" people do, merely getting a bit of support and/or tolerance at the point where we encountered the limits set by our various handicaps.

In one sense, I am privileged: I can still go into a café or restaurant without problems and without drawing attention to myself. In a museum, too, I can get around tolerably well. At the Munich Oktoberfest, though, it starts to get difficult. But what will it look like in a few months' or years' time? "Well, then you'll have to ask family, friends or neighbours to go with you," I hear you say. But maybe that's not what I want. Perhaps I'd like to be independent in the future, too, and above all not to be constantly pestering other people with my neediness. In short, I'm interested in leisure activities for people with dementia that don't require support from relatives, friends, etc., and are still as normal as possible. By "normal" I mean activities that are not intended as treatment for impairments caused by dementia, but are for general edification and recreation, without constantly reminding me about my dementia. My request to those without dementia (which I make in common with many others *with* dementia) is therefore: rejoice with us about the things we can still do, and don't complain about what we've lost, since, as a rule, you can't change it.

In the Munich Alzheimer's Society this has been done to the extent that joint activities have been organised for people with and without dementia. A particular event of this kind was on 14 July 2010: a trip for patients and family members to a golf course near Munich. Assisted by a club that aims to promote social projects, we were to spend a full day acquainting ourselves with golf – indeed, five golf instructors were waiting for us – and having an enjoyable day.

Everything went well: the weather was wonderful and the programme appealing – everything would have been perfect, had it not been for some nuances and overtones.

All day I, and others too, had the feeling that we were not being taken seriously on that golf trip. It's not at all easy to pin this feeling down onto concrete events; it was the cumulative effect of small details that led to the impression. There were, for example, the announcements made by a social worker who accompanied us, along the lines of: "Hello, just listen to me, I'm talking now. Here comes the music." Or: "Over here, everyone. Over here. Put your backpacks there, in the corner. But quickly. I said, over here, everyone." Of course, saying things like this can be explained in terms of poor manners or stress. But if it keeps happening all day, you start to wonder. To give another example: to start with, we all practised holding a golf club and tried putting the ball into the hole. This was great fun, and the golf instructors, too, seemed to take pleasure in teaching us novices a few basics. They went to a lot of trouble, even with group members who didn't understand straightaway what they were supposed to be doing with the club and ball. Everyone joined in and was supported within the range of their abilities. A small competition was planned for the afternoon. There's nothing wrong with that – one way or another, all of us need to measure ourselves in competitions or games. All of us played against one another – people with dementia and fit-as-a-fiddle relatives alike. You can imagine the outcome. To the person with dementia, their own disabilities couldn't be more obvious. Wouldn't it have been better to have two or three mixed groups playing against one another? Wasn't that the idea of "integration"?

"What's that Rohra woman whinging about now? She ought to be grateful for the great outing! Anyway, it was only a game." Is that what you were just thinking? Perhaps you're right; possibly I am finicky, ungrateful and, on top of that, a bad loser. Perhaps we people with dementia are also particularly sensitive to these nuances and can hear the grass growing everywhere because we are so torn between our wish to be treated like normal people, on the one hand, and our need for support and recognition on the other. Whatever the reason, we notice immediately if we are not being treated as adult, mature people, and I'm certain that this applies not just to those who can still express themselves verbally. Those in the more advanced stages also have a keen sense for this.

In passing let me tell you that the social worker who accompanied us to the golf course left the Munich Alzheimer's Society soon afterwards, by her own choice. I can only hope that in the meantime she has found a field of activity that suits her abilities and inclinations, and I wish her well on her path.

# TWENTY

# Why it's wrong to compare people with dementia to children

It's a commonplace belief that we people with dementia become children again. Personally, if I may say so, I feel that remarks like this are insulting, or at the very least a thoughtless reduction of reality. Describing us as children or, even worse, treating us as such, automatically deprives us of our maturity and pushes our will and our opinions into the zone of expressions of feeling that need not be taken seriously.

We are not children. We can look back on a long life with experiences and memories in which we have formed values and attitudes. Besides simple likes and dislikes, which, without question, children also have, over the course of time we have adopted a lifestyle that is far more complex than a child's. We have been able, or have had, to make decisions with far-reaching consequences: for example, choice of career, of a life partner; the decision whether or not to have children of our own, or where to live. Many of these decisions we were able to make ourselves, regardless of general conditions; we were autonomous to a large degree. Children, by contrast, live naturally in a world that is controlled by others, where a goal of childhood and youth is, precisely, to become autonomous. But why should we, who long ago attained the age of majority, want to give up our autonomy? The belief that beyond a certain point people with dementia can no longer look after themselves, and therefore need to be governed by others, is partly correct; but we don't become children because of that.

Unfortunately our own intellectual attainments are not always immediately available to us, or we can't articulate them adequately. Nevertheless, our recollections of past events are always suffused with our attitudes and values, and so we have a very clear sense of when the overall tone of present events differs from what we knew before. Without question, normal people are no different here; only *we* are not always unreservedly credited with this ability.

Don't treat us like children! Even if our behaviour or emotionality don't fully meet the expectations that you normally have of adults – since we react in a more direct manner, beyond customarily accepted social norms – we aren't behaving in a childish way! Sometimes we understand situations in a different way from you. Possibly, at times, we are disorientated, making incorrect links between the present and the past. In these situations I ask you to be kind and tolerant. Dispense with explanations that on the whole confuse us even more. Simply tell us how you understand a situation, so that we can meet on an equal footing.

# TWENTY ONE

# Things that I would like people to do when interacting with people with dementia

Living with dementia means living with either the threat or the reality of losing mental capacity, and coming to terms with that. Believe me, parting with knowledge and skills that you've gained over the course of decades is not easy. If it were only a matter of forgetting something we learnt at school – the tributaries of the Danube, the German Baltic ports or the names and succession of the presidents of Germany – then our chances in "Who Wants to Be a Millionnaire?" would be reduced, but apart from that our life would follow a (for the most part) normal course. Probably we wouldn't even notice the loss. But with the skills of daily living it's a different matter entirely: reading a town map, using one's own computer, booking a ticket on the Internet, filling in the details to make a bank transfer, etc. If you lose these skills, then, as a person with dementia, you are up against your own limits every day. Limits that weren't there before. Thus dementia is constantly perceptible and reminding you of your own impairments.

I personally would prefer not to give in to these losses without a fight, and as long as it's at all possible I'd like to manage my affairs myself. Sometimes, therefore, I need a bit more time to fill out a form; or I have to ask several times before I can understand something. I know I'm expecting a lot of you when I ask for your patience. But please don't take over if something doesn't go right first time. Of course you can do lots of things down to a T and a lot faster than we can. But if everything is done for us, even with the best of intentions, we lose our abilities. "Use it, or lose it." Just as you might forget a foreign language that you've had no occasion to use since school, the less we practice even simple actions, the faster we forget them. I do know that sometimes we are helped because people without dementia can't bear it when we're clumsy. Then, feeling ashamed on our behalf, they take over and quickly put an end to it. The embarrassing situation is over, everything's back in order – for them anyway; but I, as a person with dementia, have learnt yet again how stupid and tiresome I am. In future I'll think twice before I try to peel the lid off a portion of milk at a café. Next time maybe I'll just ask for water, although I actually prefer coffee with my cake.

We are glad to be helped, no question about that; please don't leave me fumbling for hours with the soggy biscuit that comes with a cup of coffee, but be kind enough, first, to ask if I need help. You could say something mischievous like: "I always used to struggle with this packaging too. But recently I did an evening class in 'Opening packaging for beginners'. It's been a lot better since then. Shall I show you what they taught me?" Well, you know what I mean. Although, as I write this, maybe a course really is needed, even for people who haven't got dementia?

In this case I am speaking primarily for myself, but on the basis of my conversations with others, I believe that many people with dementia think and feel the same. One of the greatest horrors of dementia lies, for me, in the gradual loss of my independence – by which I mean not so much the condition of being reliant on others, as the inability to express and implement my own wishes and needs – and at a later stage no longer being able to fend off well-meant or malicious intrusions into my privacy. As yet I can still express myself, state my needs and get them seen to. At least I have the verbal abilities for that. However, if I am not taken seriously, and am compared to a child, I am being robbed of my independence, regardless of whether I can form coherent sentences or not.

People with dementia often have the experience of other people talking about them, instead of with them.

Others have told me, for example, about situations at the doctor's, where the doctor talks to their partner about their illness – in the presence of the patient, mind you, who at that moment must be feeling more like an object than a full human being. Other very similar situations arise in advice centres, with the occupational therapist or at the hairdresser's – in fact, whenever a person with dementia has a companion with them at an encounter with a third party, and everyone is aware of the dementia.

So far I've been able to handle most of my visits to the doctor and the authorities on my own, with the advantage that then they've had to address themselves to me – which is presumably not always very easy for the other person, but they couldn't avoid it by talking about my needs to someone other than me. How it will be in future, I don't know. How long I will be able to keep on managing my own affairs is uncertain. In case I ever do need support, I already have a request: talk with me, instead of about me. Don't make decisions over the top of my head, but involve me in decisions that concern me. Explain the matter to me in a way that I can understand, instead of taking the alternative that's easier for you and making a decision behind my back.

# TWENTY TWO

# Invisible hurdles in everyday life

At events and talks I'm often asked: "How does your dementia manifest in everyday life? You still speak so well. What do you struggle with the most?" Most of all I would like to reply: "I struggle the most with food packaging. Isn't it the same for you?"

However, I restrain myself and say something like this: "What annoys me the most is my slowness. Things that used not to be a problem are a performance nowadays. Whether it's a train journey, going shopping, or an invitation to coffee, I have to plan everything exactly and think it through in advance, otherwise it goes wrong. So spontaneity is a thing of the past, and that's a pain."

And indeed, it's the many small barriers that restrict me. Take my bank, for example. Until recently, in order to withdraw money I would always go to a counter, fill in the form and receive the money. But one day I was intercepted near the entrance by a bank employee and asked what I wanted. "I'd like to withdraw some money," I told her, refraining from adding, "You haven't any sandwiches today, have you?" However, the young, enthusiastic official led me up to a grey box and said, "You can only do that at our cash machines now," pointing proudly at the contraption as if it were not a cash machine but the Minister of Finance in person.

Cash and ticket machines are a big obstacle for me. It takes me an incredibly long time to tell the machine what I want it to do. In order to buy a travel ticket, you first of all have to pick out your destination, in the right zone, from a list. But the alphabet vanished from my memory long ago. Therefore I run my finger down the list until finally I spot my destination. Tap in the number quickly; and then with an effort I fumble for the right coins. Have I already mentioned the fact that mental arithmetic and recognising coins are not my strong points? However, the machine doesn't understand this, or it's also a bit demented, since meanwhile it's forgotten the zone I selected. For me, then, it's back to the beginning.

But to return to the bank official. How was I to explain my problem to her? "Hmm, that's a nuisance, I'm not familiar with the machine," was my attempt to wriggle out of the situation. "Never mind. I'll show you. Give me your card." "Bad luck," I thought, and handed her the piece of plastic, which she took with the reverence due to a communion wafer and demanded, "Now enter your PIN number." She dismissed my objection that I didn't have one, since, she said, everyone had got one from the bank. My excuse that I had forgotten the number was shattered by the recommendation that I ask for a new one. No escape. I had to put all my cards on the table: "It won't help. I've got dementia and I can't remember any numbers, and I'm not allowed to write the PIN down either. Now, for heaven's sake, please tell me how I'm to get my money!" I didn't need to be a mind-reader. Her dismayed, mistrustful, strained expression was an open book: "Because of dementia? She's much too young to have Alzheimer's. She's having me on." Pre-empting the foreseeable discussion, I tried to explain: "I have got dementia. It's rare at my age, but it does happen. Is there really no other way than the machine?" Fortunately, there was.

# TWENTY THREE

# Conferences – Talks – Events

Following my first public appearance at "THIS MAKES SENSE!" in Stuttgart, I received a whole string of invitations to conferences and events. To some I went merely as a delegate, as, for example, to the ADI Congress in Thessaloniki. At others I was able to play an active part – say, with a talk, a contribution to a workshop or on a panel. Leafing through my appointments calendar for 2010, I can hardly believe that I'm no longer working professionally. It looks to me rather as if I'd turned dementia into a career, with scarcely a week when I'm not going somewhere on at least one day on dementia-related business. The diary entries for the big conferences alone would make one believe that I was one of those whose primary task seems to consist of attending conferences:

March 2010 Alzheimer's Disease International
    (ADI), Thessaloniki

April 2010 Dementia Care Fair, Nuremberg

May 2010 Ecumenical Church Congress, Munich

June 2010 Dementia Care, Berlin

September 2010 Dementia Europe Conference, Luxemburg

October 2010 German Alzheimer's Society Congress, Brunswick

November 2010 Conference of the German [National] Ethics Council, Hamburg

When I consider how many conferences and events on the subject of dementia are held in Germany alone in the course of a year, and then recall that people with dementia play at best a subordinate role at these, I begin to think. How can this be?

All these conferences discuss ways of providing care for people with dementia, allegedly promising therapeutic approaches are introduced, new concepts of residential care are put forward, scientific evidence presented. All for the good of us people with dementia. But we barely get a chance to speak. We aren't asked what we think about all the innovative proposals, what our ideas are, what we want for ourselves. People talk over our heads. If only for this reason, I try to be present at as many conferences as possible. I interfere wherever I can, giving a first-hand account of my experiences and making demands for the integration of people with dementia.

I would like to see a good many more people with dementia attending conferences and events on the subject. Equally desirable would be participation by people with dementia, not necessarily as active speakers, but as entirely normal members of the audience. A necessary conditon for this would be an altogether more dementia-friendly atmosphere at conferences. A slower pace would be the first step in that direction, which is to say fewer talks and workshops, and longer intervals in between. I'm convinced that most events would benefit greatly in terms of quality from such a measure. The really exciting conversations happen during the intervals between talks, in the exchanges with the other delegates. Or do you think otherwise? Just imagine fifty or more people with dementia among the audience at the next conference on dementia. Don't you think that would oblige the speakers to be more considerate in the way they talk about people with dementia? Not to mention the speed at which they speak. Any sensitive speaker might be more careful about what they said – perhaps even do without the fog that often arises from overuse of specialist vocabulary. Those would be improvements for people without dementia too.

Up to a point, organisers are getting it that participants with dementia have particular needs – so sometimes provision is made for them to rest or take time out. I saw this at the Alzheimer's Europe conference in Luxemburg, even though the organisation appeared not quite up to scratch – for example most of the organisers' staff and the conference guides didn't know where the quiet room was. It was sparsely signposted, and not very quiet, but at least someone had thought that those of us with dementia might need time out now and then. Did you know that conference delegates without dementia occasionally need time out as well? In Luxemburg I found normal conference delegates so desperate for a quiet room that they were happy to share the one for people with dementia, as if that were the natural thing to do – for when, after some searching, I finally found the quiet room, there sat a gentleman hammering on his laptop and talking loudly on his mobile phone. He was a doctor, as it turned out, using the seclusion of the room to keep track of business in his office. On my asking whether he was aware of the reason for this room, he replied, "Well, the room's empty, after all. Nobody's using it." Evidently it didn't occur to him that they weren't using it on account of the fact that he was misusing it. He couldn't be persuaded to leave, and one of the organising staff whom I had asked to back me up tersely suggested that I should report it to the organising committee.

Participation by people with dementia at events like this, whether in an active role or as members of the audience, is still very much in the early days. Therefore one shouldn't attach undue importance to the example above; but perhaps it should be seen as a reason to involve people with dementia in the planning of future events, and to take into account our expertise in respect of our own needs.

I'm pleased when an organiser gives me the opportunity to speak, so that I can address maybe 100 or more people at once. I'm just as glad to present my views in discussion groups. However, I must confess that taking part in events is not always easy for me, by which I mean not so much the mental or physical effort that goes with it, but much more the financial burden. I know it's always a bit embarrassing to talk about money in public. But, dear reader, please bear with me now.

When I'm asked to contribute to an event, in my straitened financial circumstances I'm only able to say yes if the organiser pays at least my travel and overnight expenses, which, naturally, most of them do. But it gets difficult if I have to pay travel and overnight costs in advance. It's no good at all having to wait until much later for my money, as happened after one event that I went to a month before Christmas 2010. Afterwards I called the organiser several times and asked for prompt payment, and each time I was told: "That takes time." The money was in my account at the beginning of 2011. Oh, by the way: the title of the event was "Dementia – the End of Autonomy?" To which, following my experiences with the organiser, I might reply: "No, as long as one can afford to be autonomous."

Not that I want to give you a false impression. No one has to pay me €1,000 for a 20-minute talk.

I'm happy enough with a modest reimbursement of expenses – but I just can't afford to pay up front and be out of pocket. (Just in case you want to book me for a talk…)

Considering my numerous past appearances and looking ahead to those that are planned, I sometimes ask myself: "Helga, why are you doing this to yourself?" for there are moments when it all gets a bit too much for me. On the other hand, the commitments keep me active, mentally and physically. When I remember what a deep hole I fell into when I had to give up my career, I realise how important it is to have a task to do. Perhaps this is key to overcoming dementia. Of course, having a task means something different to each person. One will find theirs in their family, another in their garden, another in sport or music. For me, it's communicating with others, with or without dementia. No matter what task someone is looking for, it can be a lifeline by which one emerges from the slough of depression. As a rule, I hesitate to give advice – but here's a piece that I'd like to offer to everyone with dementia: keep active! It may be that you have to look for new activities, because you can't do the ones that you are used to as well as you did before. But, so what? Your life is ahead of you. Don't let yourself be shunted off into the sidelines. Stand up for your rights, and remember: "Nothing about us, without us!"

# TWENTY FOUR

# Visibility and the "Dementia Card"

In a previous chapter I told you about an experience I had at my bank, and about my brave attempts to convince a bank official who believed in technology that, owing to limitations caused by dementia, I was unable to take advantage of the blessings embodied in a cash machine. One-to-one, in a small, quiet room, I could tolerate a situation of this kind. But not in the main hall of a bank, with half a dozen curious onlookers breathing down my neck. That I can do without, every bit as much as glances in the supermarket as I make my way along the shelves with my special shopping list. Since I'm no good with written shopping lists, I've taken to cutting pictures out of catalogues for the things I need most, and sticking them onto a piece of paper. Equipped with these collages, I amble along the aisles until I find the matching items – a sometimes tedious process, but one that has passed the test of time. The background to this is, of course, hidden from the other shoppers – which might explain the odd frown.

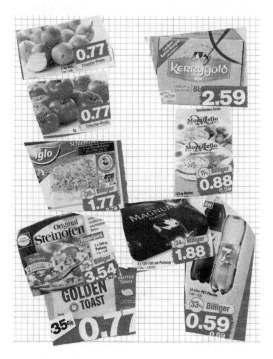

Not having our disability written all over our faces is a blessing and a curse in equal parts. I enjoy being able to walk down the street in a totally unselfconscious way, without being instantly recognised as someone with dementia. People with physical disabilities often don't have this good fortune. We, on the other hand, especially if we're on the young side, have to explain our need of support, be that in a bank, in a shop, at a ticket machine, to an authority, and so on. Every time, we hope for the slightest demonstration of understanding for our situation. Truth be told, I have to admit that in many cases I am helped in a courteous way.

In spite of everything, I find it unpleasant to have to refer to my dementia in public – which is actually a contradiction, since, on the other hand, I will go on stage and talk about it. However, the connection here is completely different. If I appear in public and talk about myself and my dementia, I am deciding what to say and what to keep to myself. In addition, I start from the assumption that the audience consists mainly of people who would like to learn something about living with dementia and are open to my point of view. In general, I then prefer to talk about my abilities and my surviving resources. I mostly gloss over my limitations and difficulties. My aim is to paint the audience a different picture of dementia. Dementia is not just decline and disintegration, and certainly not a long journey into oblivion. We are absolutely able to talk about our experience, and we also have something to say. And only we are able to describe what living with dementia is like. At events I therefore slip into the role of an expert on the internal perspective on dementia. In those moments the relationship between me as patient, and the audience as normal, is reversed. The normal people become the learners, while the patients are the ones with expertise. This makes it easy for me to talk about my dementia at public events.

It's quite different in situations where I have to justify my handicaps, where I have to explain why I need a bit more time, ask twice, or don't see straight away that a €20 note is not enough to pay a €20.10 bill. In these situations I'm surrounded by passers-by who have no understanding of dementia, and for whom dementia is synonymous with gaga or stupid. Not that anyone would openly say that to me. But if, for example, at an information desk, I indicate: "You see, I've got dementia, I can't understand that straight away," and ask to be told for the third time how to get somewhere, I can sense: "What's up with her, she's not even looking." But if it's like that for me, how must it feel to all those who don't want, or aren't able, to make their diagnosis public?

For this reason, in the Scottish Dementia Working Group people with dementia designed a card the size of a bank card, on which is written: "I have an illness called dementia. I would be glad of your help and understanding." On the reverse are a few details about the kind of support that's needed and an emergency contact address. The whole thing, bearing the official logo of the Scottish Alzheimer's Society, is a great help, according to my Scottish friends. Particularly in Scotland, much is being done to raise awareness of the "Dementia Help Card". Unfortunately, as far as I know, no comparable solution combined with effective publicity has caught on in Germany.

I possess a more or less homemade card that a Rottenburg-Stuttgart diocese worker created and handed to me, following an event at which I had been speaking on similar topics; and believe it or not, I used the card that very evening. The event, at an old people's home near Stuttgart, had lasted until late in the evening, so that I had to get the last train from Stuttgart to Munich at a quarter past ten. I was on the platform punctually, waiting for the train to arrive. Soon after the scheduled departure time the announcement "Train delayed indefinitely" appeared on the information screen, which immediately made me anxious. I looked around at the other travellers in the hope of finding someone I could tag along with, and asked if anyone else was travelling to Munich. Thus, in the end, I found a confidence-inspiring elderly gentleman with the same destination as myself. After a brief consultation we went to the information desk together. On the way we were joined by another very agitated lady. At the information desk we learned that the train's arrival would be delayed for one to two hours, on account of a personal injury. In the station's only remaining open bar the three of us whiled away the time in conversation until, around midnight, we got impatient and went back to the information desk. "There's nothing more that I can tell you. We can book you into a hotel in Stuttgart, or we can get you to Munich by taxi," was the answer to our question about what happened next. The taxi/hotel option was offered only after a discussion that ultimately involved a supervisor. At that moment I pulled out my brand new "help card" and laid it on the counter with the words: "A hotel is out of the question for me, I'm not prepared for it. I'd prefer a taxi. But it would have to take me to my front door on the edge of the city, because by the time we get to Munich Central Station there'll be no more underground or buses." Wonders never cease; they bucked up and granted us the journey by taxi, and a really friendly taxi driver landed an unexpected long-distance trip, for which he thanked us by buying us coffee at a motorway service station. And the best of it was, thanks to my new card I was spared any further embarrassment.

# TWENTY FIVE

# Mulling over my favourite topics

While working on this book, I've been intensively reviewing the past three years. It hasn't always been easy. Through talking and writing about my experiences, I've been through a lot of them all over again. Some things churned me up so much that I thought for days about things long past. However, I can't say that thinking about my more recent past has depressed and upset me. Instead, today I can see my situation more clearly, I live each day more consciously and know how to apply my energy. So it's time for me to lay memories to rest for a bit, and look towards the future.

As a result of living with dementia, there has been a critical change in the way I consider the question: "What shall I do in the future?" Before, it seemed possible to plan everything: the annual holiday, the next job, or next Christmas – everything was going to take place in the way that I intended. Even life events that are linked with big changes, such as entering retirement, could be calculated. Today it's different. I don't know how my dementia will develop, whether things will carry on the same as they have up to now, or whether I'll have to learn more quickly how to live with increasing limitations. The future now looks more like a rough sketch, and less like a concrete plan. Today I'm concerned with questions that only a few months ago had no importance:

- Will I myself notice if my mental powers decline, or will I find out from other people?

- How long will it be until I'm no longer able to make my own decisions about my life?

- Will I be able to afford to spend my last years in a home where people with dementia can find fulfilment in their lives?

- How long will I, as a person with dementia, continue to have the ability, and the candour, to quell the reticence and fear that people have around us? I am still able to approach people who don't have dementia – but for how long?

Along with these questions goes the fear of becoming totally dependent and losing my greatest resource: my ability to express myself verbally. At the same time resistance also stirs in me, since:

- I wish at all costs to persuade the media to present us, people with dementia, with all our resources, in a positive light

- it would be nice if we were able to explain at conferences that medication can ONLY be a partial support for people with dementia

- I want to have enough strength, for long enough, to fight and see the day when the limitations caused by dementia will be recognised as a disability just like other physical or mental disability

- I want the work done by family members or others in caring for us to be recognised as working time.

My dream is:

- for people with dementia to have the opportunity to do meaningful work and take on responsibilities in the Alzheimer's Societies

- that on all important committees OUR representative should speak for US – on ethics Councils, in asssociations for the disabled, on parish and town councils, in parliaments, and anywhere else where there is discussion and decision-making concerning our interests

- that there should be a portfolio for dementia within the Ministry of Health and the Ministry for Families

- that we, people with dementia, should be in solidarity, and should receive the support that WE consider necessary for this

- that we should produce our own magazine, in print or on the Internet, in which to publish our subject matter.

# Acknowledgements

My thanks to:

- my son Jens, for being together

- my friend Brigitte, for her loving companionship and empathy

- my doctor, Dr Varga, for her commitment

- my neurologist, Dr Pauls, for medical care

- my ideal escort, Prof Förstl

- my online "encouragement doctor", Dr Peter Whitehouse

- Dementia Support Stuttgart, for their collaboration

- my friend Christine Czeloth-Walther, for believing in me

- my friend Christine Bryden, for great exchanges of ideas

- my "new family" – everyone with dementia and their relatives – for their encouragement

- the star photographer Sammy Hart, for the photo he let me have

- the Munich Alzheimer's Society – first rate under its manager, Frau Zarzitzky.

My special thanks go to Dementia Support Stuttgart and its scientific officer, Falko Piest. They were the first to bring people with dementia centre stage at the conference "THIS MAKES SENSE!" Without Falko Piest's companionship, care and special commitment this wonderful book would never have been written.

Thanks to my publisher, Mabuse Verlag, and Herr Tobias Frisch for their confidence in me, and for having the courage to publish, for the first time, the thoughts and feelings of a lady with dementia!

# Afterword

A person with dementia writes a book about living with dementia. "How is that possible?" will ask the many who associate dementia with confused, completely helpless old people. That is part of the reality of people with dementia; Helga Rohra shows a different, unknown part – the early stages of dementia. She rightly deplores the fact that it is mostly the advanced stages that are presented in public, and that dementia is portrayed as an unmitigated disaster. Health professionals fall short in the way they describe dementia, since they see it from a deficit-focused angle, and far too often talk *about*, not *with*, people with dementia. Overlooking the patient's point of view results in lack of respect for the human need for esteem, autonomy, and hence a bit of normality.

Helga Rohra talks in a confident and nuanced way about her impairments, fears and coping strategies. She depicts dementia in a way that brings home the experience of it, and exposes the error in the belief that people with dementia are just passive victims of the process of cerebral decline. She addresses many problems and shortcomings in medical care and social security legislation: the Odyssey to reach a correct diagnosis; faulty or insensitive explanations and advice; bureaucratic hurdles; and the many obstacles in everyday life. She describes how anxious and depressed she was before diagnosis, and how, following an initial spell in shock after diagnosis, she got back in control of her life. She tells us where she looked for help, and above all where she found support. She has accepted the diagnosis of dementia and integrated it into her life, knows her strengths and weaknesses, and has arranged her daily living accordingly.

She provides impressive proof that people can live fulfilling lives despite dementia. Part of this is having the feeling of being taken seriously, having a purpose in life and an understanding, well-informed communal environment that helps when necessary, without being patronising. Helga Rohra, with her (not uncommon form of) dementia – Lewy Body dementia – with, at the same time, early onset, and above all her proactive way of dealing with it, is unrepresentative of the many, mostly older people, who develop dementia. She raises the bar very high, and so cannot be a yardstick for the majority of patients!

The experiences of loss that come with progression of the disease are more varied for people at the middle stage of life. But this does not alter the fact that dementia carries a high risk of stigma for young and old people alike, frequently causing isolation and exclusion and involving much suffering. It is to be hoped that more older people with dementia will also step out of the shadows and help to change the current, very negative image of dementia.

Dementia matters to all of us. We need a social climate in which people with dementia can live independently and autonomously for as long as possible, without fear, and be able to participate in social life. Current research suggests that this will not be achievable by means of medication in the foreseeable future; but with precisely the commitment and active lifestyle demonstrated by Helga Rohra, it may be. Nowadays, in our long-lived society, dementia is already normal, as one in three people develops it and many others experience the effects. All of us must make it our concern.

*Dr Elisabeth Stechl*
*Ev Geriatrie-Zentrum Berlin*
*Prof Dr Hans Förstl*
*Psychiatrische Universitätsklinik, Munich*